Managing High Blood Pressure

for Seniors

Effective Approaches for Controlling and Preventing

Hypertension to Promote Healthier Living

Sharon M. kuntz

Disclaimer

The information in this book is not intended as medical advice. Always consult with a qualified healthcare professional before making changes to your diet, exercise, or medication regimen.

Table of Contents

Introduction

Understanding the Impact of High Blood Pressure on Seniors

As we age, our bodies experience numerous changes, many of which can affect our health in significant ways. One of the most pressing issues for seniors is the management of high blood pressure, also known as hypertension. This condition, often referred to as the "silent killer," poses a unique set of challenges for older adults, making it crucial to understand and manage successfully.

High blood pressure is particularly concerning for seniors because it doesn't always appear with obvious symptoms, yet it can lead to serious health complications if left unmanaged. These consequences include heart disease, stroke, kidney failure, and even cognitive decline. The likelihood of getting hypertension rises with age, and as life expectancy continues to rise, more seniors are living with this condition. However, many are unaware of the full extent of the risks it offers or the steps they can take to mitigate these dangers.

The importance of managing high blood pressure cannot be overstated. For seniors, effective blood pressure control is not just about adding years to life; it's about adding life to years. Proper management can greatly improve quality of life, allowing seniors to maintain their freedom, engage in activities they enjoy, and avoid debilitating health issues that could otherwise limit their abilities.

This book matters because it addresses the specific needs of seniors, giving practical, evidence-based strategies to help manage high blood pressure successfully. Unlike younger people, seniors face unique challenges, such as age-related changes in blood vessels, the presence of multiple health conditions, and the potential for interactions between various medications. This guide takes these factors into account, giving tailored advice that considers the complexities of aging.

Furthermore, the book serves as a complete resource, empowering seniors with knowledge about their condition and equipping them with tools to take control of their health. It stresses the importance of a holistic approach, combining lifestyle changes, regular monitoring, and, when necessary, medication management. The goal is to help seniors make informed choices that will improve their well-being and reduce the risks associated with high blood pressure.

In addition to offering practical advice, this book also tries to dispel common myths and misconceptions about high blood pressure. Many seniors may think that hypertension is an inevitable part of aging or that there is little they can do to control it. This guide challenges those beliefs, showing that with the right knowledge and strategies, seniors can successfully manage their blood pressure and lead healthy, fulfilling lives.

Ultimately, this book matters because it provides seniors and their caregivers with the information and support they need to handle the challenges of high blood pressure. By understanding the effect of hypertension and taking proactive steps to manage it, seniors can safeguard their heart health, reduce the risk of complications, and enjoy a better quality of life in their later years. This book is more than just a guide—it's a companion on the road to better health and longevity.

How to Use This Guide

Managing high blood pressure, especially as a senior, can feel overwhelming at times. The abundance of knowledge, different treatment options, and the need to make lifestyle changes might leave you wondering where to begin. This guide is meant to be your companion on this journey, giving clear, practical advice to help you navigate the path to better health. Understanding how to use this guide successfully will ensure that you get the most out of it and can apply its lessons to your daily life.

Starting with the Basics

The first step in managing your high blood pressure is knowing what it is and how it affects your body. This guide starts by explaining the fundamentals of high blood pressure—what it is, what causes it, and why it's particularly important for seniors to manage it carefully. These chapters provide a foundation of knowledge that will help you better understand your condition and the reasons behind the suggestions that follow.

Personalized Strategies for Your Health

As you move through the guide, you'll notice that the information is tailored especially to the needs of seniors. The advice given here takes into account the unique challenges that come with aging, such as changes in metabolism, mobility, and the possibility for other health conditions that may interact with high blood pressure. Each chapter is designed to build on the last, guiding you step-by-step through the process of managing your blood pressure successfully.

This guide covers a wide range of strategies, from dietary adjustments and physical exercise to stress management and medication. The aim is to provide a comprehensive method that addresses all aspects of your health, not just your blood pressure. By following the suggestions in this book, you can build a personalized plan that fits your lifestyle, preferences, and medical needs.

Practical Tools for Daily Life

Managing high blood pressure takes consistent effort, but this guide is here to make that process easier. Throughout the book, you'll find useful tools and tips to help you incorporate healthy habits into your daily routine. For example, the parts on nutrition include meal planning tips and lists of heart-healthy foods, while the chapters on exercise offer senior-friendly workout routines that can be done at home or in your community.

In addition to lifestyle advice, this guide also stresses the importance of monitoring your blood pressure regularly. You'll learn how to measure your blood pressure at home, what the numbers mean, and when to visit your doctor. By keeping track of your success, you can see the positive impact of your efforts and make adjustments as needed.

Integrating Medical and Lifestyle Approaches

One of the key messages of this guide is that managing high blood pressure often needs a mix of medical treatment and lifestyle changes. The book provides detailed information on the different types of blood pressure medications, how they work, and potential side effects. Understanding your medicine is crucial for ensuring that you're using it effectively and avoiding interactions with other treatments.

However, medicine alone is rarely enough. That's why this guide places a strong focus on lifestyle changes that can complement your medical treatment. From reducing sodium intake to increasing physical exercise, these changes can improve the effectiveness of your medication and help you achieve better control over your blood pressure.

Navigating Challenges and Staying Motivated

No Making changes to your lifestyle and controlling a chronic condition like high blood pressure isn't always easy. There will be challenges along the way, whether it's sticking to a new diet, keeping an exercise routine, or managing stress. This guide includes methods for overcoming these obstacles, with tips on staying motivated and making gradual, sustainable changes.

Moreover, the book offers insights into how to involve your family, friends, and caregivers in your health path. Having a support system can make a big difference in your success, giving encouragement and helping you stay accountable to your goals.

Revisiting and Revising Your Plan

Your health is dynamic, and so too should be your method to managing high blood pressure. As you move through this guide and begin to apply the strategies it suggests, you'll likely find that some approaches work better for you than others. This is totally normal, and the guide encourages you to revisit and revise your plan as needed.

You may find it helpful to return to certain parts as your situation evolves. For instance, if you start a new drug, you might want to revisit the section on medication management. Or, if you're looking for ways to improve your exercise routine, the chapters on physical activity can offer new ideas.

Making This Guide Your Own

Ultimately, this guide is meant to be flexible and adaptable to your needs. You don't have to read it from cover to cover all at once. Instead, think of it as a resource that you can visit as you need it. Some readers might focus first on diet and exercise, while others might start with medication control. The key is to use the guide in a way that makes sense for you.

As you work through this book, take notes, highlight parts that resonate with you, and bookmark pages that you may want to return. The more fully you engage with the material, the more you'll get out of it.

A Journey Towards Better Health

Managing high blood pressure is a journey, and like any trip, it requires preparation, guidance, and perseverance. This guide is here to support you every step of the way, giving practical advice, proven strategies, and encouragement to help you achieve your health goals. By using this guide as your roadmap, you can handle the challenges of high blood pressure with confidence and move towards a healthier, more fulfilling life.

The Importance of Managing Blood Pressure in Your Golden Years

As we hit our golden years, maintaining good health becomes increasingly important, and managing blood pressure is a crucial aspect of that. High blood pressure, or hypertension, is a common condition among older people, but its prevalence does not make it any less serious. In fact, the risks associated with high blood pressure increase with age, making it important to keep it under control to enjoy a healthy, active life.

Why Blood Pressure Management Matters More

As we age, our bodies naturally undergo changes that can affect our circulatory system. Blood tubes lose some of their elasticity, which can make it harder for blood to flow smoothly through them.

This stiffness in the arteries can lead to increased blood pressure, putting extra strain on the heart. Over time, if high blood pressure is left unchecked, it can lead to major health issues such as heart disease, stroke, kidney damage, and even cognitive decline.

In the later stages of life, the effect of high blood pressure can be more pronounced because the body's ability to repair and recover is not as strong as it once was. What might have been a manageable condition in younger years can become more complicated and possibly dangerous if not properly addressed. This is why taking steps to manage blood pressure in your golden years is not just about avoiding complications, but also about enhancing your overall quality of life.

The Link Between High Blood Pressure and Age-Related Health Issues

High blood pressure is often called a "silent killer" because it usually doesn't cause obvious symptoms until significant damage has occurred. For seniors, the stakes are even higher, as high blood pressure is closely linked to many of the health challenges that typically arise with aging.

One of the most significant risks linked with uncontrolled high blood pressure is heart disease. The heart has to work harder to pump blood against the increased pressure in the arteries, which can lead to the thickening of the heart muscle and, finally, heart failure. Additionally, high blood pressure is a major risk factor for stroke, which occurs when the blood supply to the brain is interrupted, leading to potential paralysis, speech problems, and other long-term disabilities.

Beyond the heart and brain, high blood pressure can also hurt the kidneys, which are responsible for filtering waste from the blood. Over time, this damage can lead to chronic kidney disease, which can require dialysis or a kidney transplant in serious cases. For seniors, maintaining kidney health is especially important, as the kidneys naturally become less efficient with age.

Moreover, there is growing evidence that high blood pressure can lead to cognitive decline and dementia. The brain relies on a healthy supply of blood to work properly, and when high blood pressure disrupts this supply, it can lead to memory problems, confusion, and other symptoms associated with dementia. This makes blood pressure management not just a physical health concern, but a critical factor in keeping mental sharpness and independence as you age.

Enhancing Quality of Life Through Blood Pressure Control

Managing blood pressure properly in your golden years isn't just about avoiding serious health problems; it's also about improving your day-to-day well-being. When blood pressure is under control, you're likely to feel more energetic, experience fewer headaches, and have better general health. This allows you to stay active, engage in social activities, and enjoy your best hobbies without being held back by health concerns.

Moreover, successful blood pressure management can help preserve your independence. Many seniors value their ability to live independently, and managing blood pressure is a key factor in avoiding the health issues that could lead to dependence on others. Whether it's staying fit enough to walk to the store, travel, or simply enjoy time with family and friends, keeping your blood pressure in check plays a vital role in maintaining your autonomy.

Taking Control of Your Health

The good news is that high blood pressure is controllable, even in your golden years. By adopting healthy lifestyle habits, staying active, eating a balanced diet, and following your doctor's advice, you can take control of your blood pressure and lower your chance of complications. Regular monitoring and check-ups are also crucial, as they allow you to keep track of your progress and make changes as needed.

Medication can also be an important part of controlling high blood pressure, especially if lifestyle changes alone aren't enough. Your doctor can help you find the right medication and dosage to keep your blood pressure at a healthy level, with minimal side effects.

A Path to a Healthier Future

Managing blood pressure in your golden years is one of the most important steps you can take to protect your health and ensure a vibrant, happy life. It's about more than just numbers on a blood pressure monitor—it's about protecting your health, independence, and quality of life. By taking proactive steps to control your blood pressure, you're investing in your future, ensuring that you can enjoy all the joys and opportunities that come with this stage of life. This guide will equip you with the information and tools you need to manage your blood pressure effectively and confidently, so you can look forward to many more healthy, happy years ahead.

Chapter 1: What is High Blood Pressure?

Defining Hypertension

Hypertension, widely known as high blood pressure, is a condition where the force of blood against the walls of your arteries is consistently too high. Blood pressure is the measure of how hard your heart is working to pump blood through your blood vessels. It's a crucial function of the cardiovascular system, but when the pressure is elevated over time, it can cause damage to the arteries and lead to major health problems.

Blood pressure is represented by two numbers: systolic and diastolic pressure. The systolic number (the first and higher number) tracks the pressure in your arteries when your heart beats.

The diastolic number (the second and lower number) tracks the pressure in your arteries when your heart is at rest between beats. A normal blood pressure reading is usually around 120/80 mmHg. Hypertension is identified when these numbers are consistently higher than normal, indicating that your heart and arteries are under excessive strain.

How Blood Pressure is Measured

Blood pressure is recorded using a device called a sphygmomanometer, often referred to as a blood pressure cuff. During the measurement, the cuff is wrapped around your upper arm and inflated to limit blood flow in your arteries. As the cuff slowly deflates, a healthcare professional or an automated device listens for the sound of your blood starting to flow again. The first sound heard is the systolic pressure, and when the sound disappears, the diastolic pressure is noted.

Blood pressure readings can change throughout the day and can be influenced by various factors such as stress, physical activity, and even the time of day. That's why it's important to measure your blood pressure regularly and under uniform conditions to get an accurate picture of your cardiovascular health.

For seniors, home monitoring is particularly helpful because it allows you to track your blood pressure over time in a familiar setting, which can lead to more accurate readings. It's also important to follow proper technique when measuring your blood pressure at home, such as sitting quietly for a few minutes before taking the number, keeping your arm at heart level, and using a properly fitting cuff.

The Different Stages of High Blood Pressure

High blood pressure is categorized into different stages based on the severity of the disease. These stages help doctors decide the best course of treatment and management. The stages are:

1. Elevated Blood Pressure: This is when blood pressure readings regularly fall between 120-129 systolic and less than 80 diastolic. Although not yet classified as hypertension, elevated blood pressure is a warning sign that you're at risk of getting high blood pressure if no action is taken to lower it.

2. Stage 1 Hypertension: Stage 1 is described as a systolic pressure of 130-139 mmHg or a diastolic pressure of 80-89 mmHg. At this time, lifestyle changes such as improving diet, increasing

physical activity, and reducing stress may be recommended, along with possible medication based on your overall health and risk factors.

3. Stage 2 Hypertension: This stage is diagnosed when your blood pressure regularly measures at or above 140/90 mmHg. Stage 2 hypertension typically needs a combination of lifestyle changes and medication to control. At this stage, the chance of complications like heart disease, stroke, and kidney damage increases significantly.

4. Hypertensive Crisis: This is a severe increase in blood pressure that needs immediate medical attention, generally defined as a systolic pressure over 180 mmHg or a diastolic pressure over 120 mmHg. A hypertensive crisis can cause damage to your organs and is a medical emergency. Symptoms may include severe headaches, shortness of breath, nosebleeds, or nervousness. If

you experience any of these symptoms, it's important to seek emergency care quickly.

Understanding the different stages of high blood pressure helps you and your healthcare provider tailor your treatment plan to your individual needs. By catching and managing high blood pressure early, you can reduce the risk of serious health complications and maintain a better quality of life.

Chapter 2: Causes and Risk Factors

Age-Related Changes in Blood Pressure

As we grow older, our bodies experience numerous physiological changes, and among the most critical are those affecting our cardiovascular system. These changes, which include the stiffening of blood vessels and alterations in heart function, significantly add to the increased risk of high blood pressure (hypertension) in seniors. Understanding these age-related changes is important for managing blood pressure effectively as we age.

One of the main changes that occur with age is the stiffening of the arteries, a condition known as arteriosclerosis. In our youth, arteries are usually flexible and elastic, allowing them to expand and contract easily with each heartbeat, facilitating smooth blood flow throughout the body. However, as we age, the walls of these vessels lose some of their elasticity, becoming more rigid. This loss of flexibility makes it harder for blood to flow easily, leading to an increase in blood pressure. The stiffer the arteries, the higher the pressure needed to push blood through them, resulting in hypertension.

For example, imagine a garden hose. When the hose is new and flexible, water runs through it easily, even at lower pressures. However, as the hose ages and becomes brittle, more power is needed to push the same amount of water through it. Similarly, as our vessels stiffen with age, the heart has to work harder to pump blood, which raises blood pressure.

In addition to the stiffening of the arteries, the heart itself sees changes as we age. The heart muscle can become thicker—a disease known as left ventricular hypertrophy—which reduces the efficiency of the heart's ability to pump blood. This thickening happens as a response to the increased workload placed on the heart by stiffened arteries. While this adaptation helps the heart handle the increased pressure temporarily, it can lead to long-term problems, including heart failure and persistent hypertension.

Moreover, the kidneys, which play a crucial role in regulating blood pressure by controlling fluid balance and salt levels in the body, may also become less efficient as we age. The kidneys' ability to filter blood and excrete waste products lessens over time, which can lead to an accumulation of fluid and salt in the body. This retention increases blood volume and, ultimately, blood pressure. As kidney function declines, the risk of developing hypertension rises, making regular monitoring and management of blood pressure important for older adults.

Genetic Factors and Family History

While age-related changes are a significant risk factor for hypertension, genetics also plays a crucial part in determining an individual's susceptibility to high blood pressure. If you have a family history of hypertension, you are more likely to develop the condition yourself, suggesting a strong genetic predisposition.

Genetics can affect how your body regulates blood pressure in several ways. For instance, some people may inherit genes that affect how their kidneys handle sodium, leading to greater salt retention and, consequently, higher blood pressure. Others may have a genetic predisposition that affects the sensitivity of their blood vessels to certain hormones that control blood pressure, making them more prone to hypertension.

Understanding your family history is important for managing blood pressure effectively. If hypertension runs in your family, it's important to take proactive steps to check and control your blood pressure. This may include adopting a healthier lifestyle, such as keeping a balanced diet, engaging in regular physical exercise, and avoiding smoking and excessive alcohol consumption. Additionally, regular blood pressure checks can help discover any increases early, allowing for timely intervention.

For example, if both of your parents had high blood pressure, you are at a higher chance of developing the condition as well. In such cases, it would be smart to start monitoring your blood pressure regularly, even if you're still in your 30s or 40s. By catching any signs of hypertension early, you can work with your healthcare provider to build a plan to manage your blood pressure and reduce your risk of complications.

Lifestyle Contributors: Diet, Exercise, and Stress

While age and genetics are factors beyond our control, lifestyle choices are among the most important and controllable contributors to high blood pressure. Diet, physical activity, and stress management all play important roles in either increasing or decreasing your chance of developing hypertension.

Diet: The foods you eat have a direct effect on your blood pressure. Diets high in sodium (salt) are especially harmful because sodium causes your body to retain water, which increases blood volume and, consequently, blood pressure. The American Heart Association recommends that adults consume no more than 2,300 milligrams of sodium per day, with an ideal limit of 1,500 milligrams for most adults, especially those with high blood pressure.

However, the average sodium intake in many countries exceeds these guidelines, leading to widespread cases of hypertension.

Conversely, diets rich in fruits, veggies, whole grains, and low-fat dairy products can help lower blood pressure. The DASH (Dietary Approaches to Stop Hypertension) diet is specifically meant to reduce blood pressure by emphasizing these healthy food choices and reducing salt intake. The DASH diet supports the consumption of foods that are high in potassium, calcium, and magnesium—nutrients that help control blood pressure.

For example, replacing processed foods, which are often high in sodium, with fresh fruits and vegetables can greatly reduce your sodium intake and lower your blood pressure. Additionally, adding foods like bananas, spinach, and yogurt into your diet can provide the potassium, calcium, and magnesium needed to support healthy blood pressure levels.

Exercise: Regular physical exercise is another crucial factor in managing blood pressure. Exercise improves the heart, making it more efficient at pumping blood. This efficiency lowers the pressure on your arteries, helping to keep your blood pressure in a healthy range. Lack of exercise, on the other hand, adds to weight gain, which increases the risk of high blood pressure.

Even moderate activities like walking, swimming, or gardening can have a positive effect on your blood pressure. The key is consistency—engaging in physical exercise regularly, rather than sporadically, is what makes the difference. The American Heart Association advises at least 150 minutes of moderate-intensity aerobic exercise or 75 minutes of vigorous-intensity activity each week for adults. Additionally, adding strength training exercises at least twice a week can further support heart health and blood pressure management.

For instance, if you're not used to exercise, starting with a daily 30-minute walk can help lower your blood pressure over time. As your fitness level improves, you can gradually increase the intensity or length of your workouts, further enhancing the benefits.

Stress: Chronic stress is a major contributor to high blood pressure. When you're stressed, your body releases hormones like adrenaline and cortisol, which briefly increase blood pressure by causing your heart to beat faster and your blood vessels to constrict. While this reaction is normal in short bursts, chronic stress can lead to sustained high blood pressure, increasing the risk of heart disease and stroke.

Learning how to manage stress is important for controlling blood pressure. Techniques such as deep breathing exercises, meditation, and mindfulness can help calm the nervous system and lower stress levels. Additionally, engaging in hobbies, spending time with loved ones, and ensuring you get enough sleep can all help to better stress management.

For example, practicing awareness meditation for just 10 minutes a day can help lower your stress levels and, in turn, reduce your blood pressure. Mindfulness involves focusing on the present moment, watching your thoughts and feelings without judgment, and breathing deeply to promote relaxation. Over time, this practice can help you build a more resilient response to stress, reducing its effect on your blood pressure.

Medication and Health Conditions Impacting Blood Pressure

In addition to lifestyle factors, certain medications and underlying health problems can directly influence your blood pressure. Understanding how these factors interact with your body is important for effective blood pressure management.

Medication: Some medicines can raise blood pressure as a side effect. These include certain pain medicines, such as nonsteroidal anti-inflammatory drugs (NSAIDs), decongestants, birth control pills, and even some antidepressants. If you're taking medication that affects your blood pressure, it's important to share this with your doctor. They may adjust your dosage or offer alternative treatments to mitigate the impact on your blood pressure.

For example, if you have arthritis and regularly take NSAIDs to manage pain, you might notice a rise in your blood pressure. In such cases, your doctor may suggest alternative pain management strategies, such as physical therapy or acetaminophen, which does not have the same effect on blood pressure.

Health Conditions: Several health conditions can add to the development or worsening of high blood pressure. For instance, diabetes, heart disease, and sleep apnea are closely linked to hypertension.

Diabetes changes how your body handles insulin and glucose, leading to damage to blood vessels, which in turn can cause high blood pressure. Managing diabetes through medication, diet, and exercise is important to prevent hypertension or control it if you already have it.

Kidney disease impairs the kidneys' ability to manage blood pressure by controlling fluid balance. When the kidneys are damaged, they may fail to excrete extra salt and fluid, leading to increased blood volume and higher blood pressure. Treating kidney disease and managing your fluid and salt diet can help control blood pressure.

Sleep apnea is a disease where breathing stops and starts during sleep, leading to sudden drops in blood oxygen levels. This can cause the release of stress hormones that increase heart rate and constrict blood vessels, causing spikes in blood pressure. Treating sleep apnea, often through the use of a continuous positive airway pressure (CPAP) machine, can help lower blood pressure.

For example, if you have sleep apnea and are experiencing high blood pressure, using a CPAP machine at night can help keep steady breathing and oxygen levels, reducing the strain on your cardiovascular system and lowering your blood pressure.

High blood pressure is a complex disease influenced by various factors, including age-related changes, genetics, lifestyle choices, medications, and underlying health conditions. Understanding these causes and risk factors is essential for effective blood pressure management, especially as we age.

By being aware of the changes that occur in our bodies as we age, the role of genetics, and the effect of lifestyle choices, we can take proactive steps to monitor and control our blood pressure. Additionally, understanding how certain medications and health conditions affect blood pressure allows for a more tailored approach to managing this condition.

Taking Action: A Summary of Key Strategies

1. Regular Monitoring: Make blood pressure checks a regular part of your health care. Whether you measure your blood pressure at home or have it checked during regular doctor visits, staying informed about your blood pressure levels is crucial for early detection and intervention.

2. Adopting a Heart-Healthy Diet: Follow the DASH diet or a similar heart-healthy eating plan that emphasizes fruits, veggies, whole grains, and low-fat dairy products. Reduce your sodium intake and incorporate foods rich in potassium, calcium, and magnesium to help control blood pressure.

3. Engaging in Regular Physical Activity: Aim for at least 150 minutes of moderate-intensity exercise each week. Choose activities that you enjoy and that fit your fitness level, and make physical exercise a regular part of your routine.

4. Managing Stress: Incorporate stress-reducing methods such as deep breathing, meditation, and mindfulness into your daily life. Ensure you get enough sleep and participate in hobbies and social activities that help you relax.

5. Understanding Medication and Health Conditions: If you're taking medication, be aware of its possible effects on your blood pressure. Work with your healthcare provider to change your treatment plan if necessary. Manage underlying health problems such as diabetes, kidney disease, and sleep apnea to help control your blood pressure.

6. Maintaining a Healthy Weight: If you're overweight, losing even a small amount of weight can greatly lower your blood pressure. Focus on sustainable weight loss strategies that include a balanced diet and regular physical exercise.

Chapter 3: Symptoms and Complication

Recognizing the Silent Symptoms

High blood pressure, often called the "silent killer," is a problem that can go unnoticed for years because it usually doesn't cause obvious symptoms. Many people with high blood pressure feel perfectly fine and only find their condition during a routine check-up or after a major health issue arises.

This lack of symptoms is what makes high blood pressure especially dangerous—without regular tracking, you might not realize you have a problem until it has already caused significant damage to your health.

In some cases, when blood pressure hits extremely high levels, people may experience symptoms such as severe headaches, nosebleeds, shortness of breath, or feelings of anxiety. However, these symptoms are rare and often appear only when blood pressure has hit a dangerously high level, which is considered a medical emergency. For most people, the effects of high blood pressure build slowly over time, quietly damaging the heart, blood vessels, and other organs without any warning signs.

Short-Term and Long-Term Health Risks

Although high blood pressure may not cause instant symptoms, the risks involved with it are very real. In the short run, unchecked high blood pressure puts extra strain on your heart and blood vessels. This greater strain can lead to the thickening of the heart muscle, making it harder for the heart to pump blood effectively. Over time, this can result in heart failure, where the heart can no longer meet the body's needs.

The long-term health risks of high blood pressure are even more dangerous. Persistent high blood pressure can damage the arteries, making them less flexible and more prone to the buildup of fatty deposits. This condition, known as atherosclerosis, narrows the arteries and restricts blood flow, increasing the risk of heart attack and stroke.

In addition to harming the heart and arteries, high blood pressure can also harm other organs, especially the kidneys. The kidneys rely on healthy blood vessels to clear waste from the blood. When high blood pressure damages these vessels, it can lead to kidney disease or even kidney failure, which may require dialysis or a kidney donor. Moreover, high blood pressure can affect the eyes, leading to eyesight problems or even blindness, and it can also cause sexual dysfunction by reducing blood flow to the reproductive systems.

The Connection Between High Blood Pressure and Heart Disease, Stroke, and Kidney Problems

The most dangerous complications of high blood pressure are closely linked to three major health concerns: heart disease, stroke, and kidney problems. Understanding these connections is important for understanding the importance of managing blood pressure effectively.

1. Heart Disease: High blood pressure is one of the main risk factors for heart disease, which is the number one cause of death worldwide. When blood pressure is constantly high, it causes the heart to work harder, which can lead to the thickening of the heart muscle, especially the left ventricle. This disease, known as left ventricular hypertrophy, increases the chance of heart attack, heart failure, and sudden cardiac death. Additionally, high blood pressure can add to the development of coronary artery disease, where the arteries that give blood to the heart become narrowed or blocked, leading to chest pain (angina) or a heart attack.

2. Stroke: Stroke happens when the blood flow to the brain is interrupted, either by a blocked artery (ischemic stroke) or a burst blood vessel (hemorrhagic stroke). High blood pressure is the most important risk factor for both types of stroke. By hurting and weakening the blood vessels in the brain, high blood pressure makes them more likely to burst or become blocked. A stroke can lead to severe disability or death, and for those who survive, the healing process can be long and difficult, often involving physical therapy and other forms of rehabilitation.

3. Kidney Problems: The kidneys play an important part in regulating blood pressure by controlling the amount of fluid in the body and filtering out waste products from the blood. High blood pressure damages the small blood vessels in the kidneys, lowering their ability to work properly. This can lead to chronic kidney disease, a situation where the kidneys gradually lose their ability to filter blood successfully. If left untreated, chronic kidney disease can move to kidney failure, needing dialysis or a kidney transplant. Additionally, high blood pressure can increase the progression of kidney disease in people who already have conditions such as diabetes.

High blood pressure is a problem that often goes unnoticed, but its effects on the body can be deadly. By recognizing the silent nature of hypertension and learning the short-term and long-term health risks it poses, you can take proactive steps to manage your blood pressure and protect your health. The strong connections between high blood pressure and serious conditions like heart disease, stroke, and kidney problems show the value of regular monitoring and effective management. By staying informed and taking action, you can reduce the chance of these complications and keep a healthier, more satisfying life.

Chapter 4: Getting Diagnosed

How Blood Pressure is Diagnosed

Diagnosing high blood pressure is a straightforward process that mainly involves measuring your blood pressure using a simple, non-invasive test. This test can be done at a doctor's office, a store, or even at home using a personal blood pressure monitor. The goal is to determine whether your blood pressure is within a healthy level or if it's elevated, indicating hypertension.

High blood pressure is usually diagnosed based on multiple readings taken over time. Since blood pressure can fluctuate throughout the day due to various factors such as stress, physical exercise, and even the time of day, a single reading isn't enough to make a diagnosis. Your healthcare provider will likely take several measurements at different times or ask you to watch your blood pressure at home over a period of days or weeks to get an accurate assessment.

What to Expect During a Blood Pressure Test

When you have your blood pressure checked, you'll usually sit in a chair with your arm resting on a table at heart level. The healthcare worker or technician will wrap a cuff around your upper arm. This cuff is linked to a device called a sphygmomanometer, which measures the pressure in your arteries.

Here's what happens during the test

1. Cuff Inflation: The cuff is expanded by either a hand pump or an automatic device until it tightens around your arm. This temporarily stops the blood flow in your artery.

2. Measurement: As the cuff slowly deflates, the healthcare provider will listen to the sound of your blood starting to flow again using a stethoscope, or an automated machine will identify the flow. The first sound heard is the systolic pressure, and when the sound stops, the diastolic pressure is recorded.

3. Recording the Results: The results are given as two numbers. For example, a blood pressure reading might be 120/80 mmHg, where the first number (120) represents the systolic pressure and the second number (80) represents the diastolic pressure.

The test is quick and painless, typically taking just a few minutes. It's important to stay still and relaxed during the measurement, as talking or moving can affect the reading. In some cases, the healthcare provider may take repeated readings in both arms to ensure accuracy.

Understanding Your Blood Pressure Numbers

Blood pressure readings are stated as two numbers, one over the other, measured in millimeters of mercury (mmHg). The two numbers describe different aspects of how blood moves through your arteries:

Systolic Pressure: The top number in a blood pressure result is the systolic pressure. It measures the pressure in your arteries when your heart beats and pumps blood. This number is important because it shows how much pressure your blood is exerting against the artery walls during the most active phase of your heart's cycle.

Diastolic Pressure: The bottom number is the diastolic pressure, which measures the pressure in your vessels when your heart is at rest between beats. This number shows how much pressure your blood exerts against the artery walls when the heart is not actively pumping.

Here's what the numbers mean

1. Normal Blood Pressure: A normal reading is usually considered to be around 120/80 mmHg or lower. If your numbers fall within this range, your blood pressure is considered good.

2. Elevated Blood Pressure: If your systolic pressure is between 120-129 mmHg and your diastolic pressure is less than 80 mmHg, you have elevated blood pressure. This is not yet hypertension, but it's a sign that you need to take steps to lower your blood pressure to keep it from progressing.

3. Stage 1 Hypertension: This is identified when your systolic pressure is between 130-139 mmHg or your diastolic pressure is between 80-89 mmHg. At this stage, lifestyle changes and probably medication are recommended to bring your blood pressure down.

4. Stage 2 Hypertension: Stage 2 is described by a systolic pressure of 140 mmHg or higher or a diastolic pressure of 90 mmHg or higher. This stage often needs a combination of medication and lifestyle adjustments to control the problem.

5. Hypertensive Crisis: If your blood pressure readings suddenly exceed 180/120 mmHg, you may be having a hypertensive crisis, which requires instant medical attention. Symptoms like severe headache, chest pain, or shortness of breath may accompany this disease.

Understanding these numbers is important for managing your health. Regular monitoring can help you keep track of any changes in your blood pressure and take action before it leads to more major complications. If your readings regularly fall into the elevated or hypertensive range, it's crucial to work with your healthcare provider to develop a plan to lower your blood pressure and reduce your risk of heart disease, stroke, and other related conditions.

Getting your blood pressure diagnosed is an easy but vital step in protecting your health. By understanding what happens during a blood pressure test and learning how to interpret the results, you can take an active part in managing your blood pressure and preventing serious health issues. Regular monitoring and knowledge of your blood pressure numbers are key to keeping good cardiovascular health and ensuring that any issues are caught and addressed early.

Chapter 5: Choosing the Right Blood Pressure Monitor

When it comes to managing high blood pressure, having a reliable blood pressure monitor at home is important. With so many options available, finding the right one can feel overwhelming, but it doesn't have to be. The first step is to decide whether you want an upper-arm monitor or a wrist monitor. Upper-arm monitors are usually more accurate and are recommended by most healthcare professionals. They consist of a cuff that wraps around your upper arm and a monitor that shows your readings.

When choosing a monitor, consider the following factors:

1. Accuracy: Look for a monitor that has been clinically confirmed for accuracy. This ensures that the numbers you get are reliable and consistent with what you would receive at a doctor's office.

2. Ease of Use: The monitor should be easy to use, with clear directions. Some models have large digital displays, which are helpful if you have vision problems. Automated devices that inflate the cuff and take readings with just the push of a button are usually the most user-friendly.

3. Cuff Size: The cuff size is important for getting an accurate reading. Most monitors come with a standard-sized cuff, but if your arm is bigger or smaller than average, make sure to get a cuff that fits properly. A poorly fitted cuff can give inaccurate readings.

4. Memory and Data Storage: Many modern monitors can store multiple readings for one or more people, which is helpful if you want to track your blood pressure over time or share the data with your healthcare provider. Some even have Bluetooth features, allowing you to sync your readings with a smartphone app.

5. Price: While it's important to find a monitor that fits your budget, remember that accuracy and dependability are more important than cost. There are many affordable choices that still offer good performance.

How to Measure Blood Pressure at Home Accurately

Taking your blood pressure at home can give you a more accurate picture of your heart health since it matches your typical environment.

However, it's important to measure it properly to ensure the readings are reliable.

Here's how to measure your blood pressure at home accurately:

1. Prepare Yourself: Before getting a reading, avoid smoking, caffeine, or exercise for at least 30 minutes, as these can affect your blood pressure. Sit quietly for five minutes before starting. Make sure your bladder is empty, as a full bladder can also raise your blood pressure.

2. Proper Positioning: Sit in a comfortable chair with your back supported and both feet flat on the floor. Your arm should be held on a flat surface, with the cuff at heart level. Rest your arm on a table or the armrest of a chair to keep it in the right position.

3. Apply the Cuff Correctly: Wrap the cuff snugly around your upper arm, about an inch above the bend of your elbow. Ensure there are no clothes between your skin and the cuff. The cuff should be level with your heart for the most accurate reading.

4. Stay Still and Quiet: Press the start button on your monitor, and stay still and quiet while the machine inflates the cuff and takes the reading. Moving or talking during the measurement can affect the readings.

5. Take Multiple Readings: For accuracy, it's a good idea to take two or three readings, one minute apart, and record the average of the readings. This helps account for any fluctuations and gives a more accurate measure of your blood pressure.

6. Time of Day: Try to take your readings at the same time each day, as blood pressure can change throughout the day. Morning and evening readings are often suggested.

Keeping a Blood Pressure Log: What to Record

Keeping a blood pressure log is an effective way to track your health and share information with your healthcare provider. A log helps you spot trends, see how your blood pressure changes over time, and determine how well your treatment plan is working.

Here's what to record in your blood pressure log

1. Date and Time: Always note the date and time of each reading. This helps track how your blood pressure changes throughout the day and from day to day.

2. Blood Pressure Readings: Record both the systolic (top number) and diastolic (bottom number) readings. For example, you might write 120/80 mmHg.

3. Heart Rate: Some monitors also measure your heart rate, which can provide extra information about your cardiovascular health. Record your pulse if your monitor gives this data.

4. Position and Arm Used: Note whether you were sitting or lying down during the reading, as well as which arm you used. It's usually recommended to use the same arm each time for consistency.

5. Notes on Conditions: Record any factors that might have changed the reading, such as feeling stressed, having just exercised, or taking medication. Also, note any symptoms you may be having, such as dizziness or headache.

6. Medications and Dosages: If you're taking medication for high blood pressure or other conditions, note the name and dosage, as well as the time you took it related to your blood pressure reading. This helps track how your medication changes your blood pressure.

7. Comments or Observations: Include any other observations, such as dietary changes, new physical hobbies, or changes in sleep patterns. These can help you and your doctor understand the factors affecting your blood pressure.

By carefully keeping a log, you'll have a valuable tool for managing your blood pressure. This record can be shared with your healthcare provider, letting them make informed decisions about your treatment plan and any necessary adjustments.

Home monitoring is a strong tool in managing high blood pressure. By choosing the right monitor, learning how to take accurate readings, and keeping a thorough log, you can take charge of your health. These steps not only provide you with instant feedback but also give your healthcare provider the information needed to tailor your treatment plan effectively.

Regular monitoring, combined with professional advice, can help you keep better control over your blood pressure and improve your overall well-being.

Chapter 6: Regular Check-Ups

The Importance of Routine Doctor Visits

Routine doctor visits are a crucial part of controlling high blood pressure, especially as we age. These regular check-ups serve as the foundation for effective healthcare, ensuring that any changes in your health are identified early and addressed quickly. For individuals with high blood pressure, or those at risk, these visits can be life-saving by helping to avoid serious complications such as heart disease, stroke, and kidney failure.

One of the main reasons routine visits are so important is that high blood pressure often doesn't cause noticeable symptoms. Without regular monitoring, you might not even know your blood pressure is elevated. By seeing your doctor regularly, you give them the opportunity to measure your blood pressure, review your overall health, and make any necessary changes to your treatment plan.

During these visits, your doctor can also assess how well your present blood pressure management strategies are working. If your blood pressure remains high despite your efforts, they can recommend changes, whether that means adjusting your medication, suggesting lifestyle modifications, or requesting additional tests to rule out underlying conditions. Early detection of problems allows for timely intervention, which can greatly reduce the chance of serious health issues down the line.

Routine doctor visits are also important for staying on top of other health problems that can affect blood pressure, such as diabetes, high cholesterol, and obesity. These conditions often require their own treatments, and managing them properly can help lower your blood pressure as well. Your doctor will consider the whole picture of your health during these visits, ensuring that all parts of your well-being are addressed.

In addition to monitoring your physical health, routine visits provide a chance to discuss any concerns or questions you might have about your treatment or condition. It's important to speak openly with your doctor about how you're feeling, any side effects you're experiencing from medication, or any difficulties you're having in following your treatment plan. This conversation helps your doctor tailor your care to your individual needs and ensures you're on the best path to managing your blood pressure.

Furthermore, these visits offer a chance to review and update your medicine. As our bodies change over time, the effectiveness of certain medicines can also change. Your doctor can evaluate whether your current prescription is still the best choice for you or if it's time to explore other medicines. They can also check for interactions between any new medications and those you're already taking, lowering the risk of adverse effects.

Routine doctor visits also allow for important screenings and tests that can spot potential complications early. For example, regular blood tests can track kidney function, cholesterol levels, and blood sugar levels, all of which are closely linked to high blood pressure. If any of these tests show problems, your doctor can take steps to address them before they become more serious.

Finally, building a strong relationship with your healthcare provider through regular visits helps build trust and mutual understanding. When you see your doctor regularly, they become more familiar with your medical background, your preferences, and your goals. This familiarity makes it easier for them to provide personalized care that aligns with your wants and lifestyle, increasing the likelihood of successful treatment outcomes.

In summary, routine doctor visits are important for managing high blood pressure and maintaining overall health. These visits allow early detection of issues, ensure your treatment plan remains effective, and provide a platform for open communication with your healthcare provider. By making regular check-ups a goal, you can take proactive steps to protect your health, prevent complications, and live a longer, healthier life.

Chapter 7: Nutrition and Diet

The DASH Diet: Eating for Better Blood Pressure

The DASH diet, which stands for Dietary Approaches to Stop Hypertension, is one of the most successful eating plans for managing high blood pressure. It's specifically meant to help lower blood pressure by focusing on foods that are rich in nutrients like potassium, calcium, and magnesium, while also being low in sodium, saturated fat, and added sugars. By following the DASH diet, you can greatly reduce your blood pressure and improve your overall heart health.

The DASH diet stresses fruits, vegetables, whole grains, lean proteins, and low-fat dairy products.

These foods are not only nutrient-dense but also help keep your blood vessels healthy, reduce inflammation, and avoid the buildup of cholesterol in your arteries. By incorporating more of these foods into your daily meals, you can create a balanced diet that supports your blood pressure control efforts.

One of the key perks of the DASH diet is its flexibility. It's not a rigid plan but rather a guideline that encourages healthier food decisions. For instance, instead of grabbing for a bag of chips, you might opt for a handful of unsalted nuts or a piece of fruit. Over time, these small changes can lead to major improvements in your blood pressure and overall well-being.

Sodium: How Much is Too Much?

Sodium plays a major role in regulating blood pressure, and consuming too much can lead to hypertension. Sodium causes the body to retain water, which increases the amount of blood in your bloodstream and, consequently, the pressure on your blood vessels. Therefore, it's crucial to watch and limit your sodium intake, especially if you have high blood pressure.

The American Heart Association suggests that most adults should consume no more than 2,300 milligrams of sodium per day, with an ideal limit of 1,500 milligrams for those with high blood pressure. However, the average person often consumes much more, mainly due to processed foods, restaurant meals, and added salt.

Reducing salt intake starts with reading food labels carefully. Processed foods, canned goods, and frozen meals are often loaded with sodium, so it's important to choose low-sodium or no-salt-added versions whenever possible. Cooking at home gives you more control over the amount of salt in your food, and you can experiment with herbs and spices to improve flavor without relying on salt.

In addition to cutting back on processed foods, it's also wise to be aware of the salt you add during cooking and at the table. Gradually lowering the amount of salt you use can help retrain your taste buds to enjoy foods with less sodium. Over time, you'll find that you don't miss the extra salt, and your blood pressure will thank you for it.

Foods to Include and Avoid

When it comes to handling high blood pressure, the foods you choose to include in your diet are just as important as those you avoid. The DASH diet offers a great framework for making these choices.

Foods to Include:

Fruits and veggies: Aim for at least five servings of fruits and veggies each day. These foods are rich in potassium, which helps balance the effects of sodium and lowers blood pressure. Fresh, frozen, or canned fruits and vegetables (without added salt) are all good choices.

- Whole Grains: Foods like oatmeal, brown rice, whole wheat bread, and quinoa are excellent sources of fiber and help keep healthy blood pressure levels. Whole grains also help keep you full, which can aid in weight control.

- Lean nutrients: Include lean meats like chicken and turkey, as well as plant-based nutrients like beans, lentils, and tofu. These foods are low in fatty fat, which is important for heart health.

- Low-Fat Dairy: Low-fat or fat-free milk, yogurt, and cheese provide calcium, which is important for blood pressure control. Choose types with no added sugars to keep your diet as heart-healthy as possible.

- Nuts, Seeds, and Legumes: These foods are packed with nutrients like calcium and healthy fats. Just be sure to choose unsalted varieties to keep your sodium diet in check.

Foods to Avoid:

Processed Foods: These are often high in salt, unhealthy fats, and added sugars. This includes things like deli meats, packaged snacks, and fast food. Opt for whole, raw foods whenever possible.

- Sugary Beverages: Drinks like soda, sweetened coffee, and energy drinks can add to weight gain and increase your risk of high blood pressure. Water, herbal teas, and sparkling water with a splash of lemon or lime are healthier options.

- Red Meat and Full-Fat Dairy: These foods are high in saturated fat, which can raise your cholesterol levels and increase your risk of heart disease. Choose leaner cuts of meat and lower-fat dairy items instead.

- Alcohol: While reasonable alcohol consumption may not harm some people, excessive drinking can raise your blood pressure. If you drink alcohol, do so in moderation—this usually means no more than one drink per day for women and two for men.

Hydration and Blood Pressure: The Role of Water

Staying properly hydrated is an often-overlooked part of managing blood pressure. Water plays a crucial role in keeping the balance of fluids in your body, which is important for normal blood pressure. When you're dehydrated, your body holds onto sodium to spare water, which can lead to an increase in blood pressure.

To stay refreshed, it's important to drink water throughout the day. Most people should aim for about eight 8-ounce glasses of water per day, though individual needs can vary based on factors like activity level, climate, and general health. If you're unsure how much water you need, your healthcare provider can offer personalized advice.

In addition to plain water, you can also stay hydrated with herbal teas, and water-rich fruits and veggies, such as cucumbers, oranges, and melons. However, it's best to avoid sugary drinks and excessive coffee, as these can lead to dehydration and negatively impact your blood pressure.

Drinking enough water not only helps keep healthy blood pressure but also supports overall cardiovascular health, improves energy levels, and aids digestion. By making hydration a goal, you can support your efforts to manage high blood pressure and enjoy better health overall.

Nutrition plays a central part in managing high blood pressure. By following the DASH diet, limiting sodium intake, choosing the right foods, and staying hydrated, you can take major steps toward lowering your blood pressure and improving your overall health. These dietary changes, combined with regular monitoring and professional advice, form a strong basis for managing high blood pressure and living a healthier, more fulfilling life.

Chapter 8 : Physical Activity

The Benefits of Exercise for Seniors

Exercise is one of the most effective ways to manage high blood pressure, especially for seniors. Regular physical activity strengthens the heart, allowing it to pump blood more efficiently and with less effort. This lessens the force on your arteries and lowers your blood pressure. Beyond its direct effect on blood pressure, exercise also offers a wide range of other health benefits, contributing to overall well-being and a higher quality of life.

For seniors, exercise can improve cardiovascular health, increase muscle strength, and boost flexibility and balance. This combination helps prevent falls and other injuries, which are regular concerns as we age. Regular exercise also supports mental health, lowering symptoms of anxiety and sadness while improving cognitive function. Many seniors find that staying active helps them keep independence longer, allowing them to continue doing the things they enjoy with fewer limitations.

Another important benefit of exercise for seniors is weight control. Being overweight is a significant risk factor for high blood pressure, and regular physical activity helps keep a healthy weight by burning calories and building muscle.

Even modest weight loss can have a substantial effect on lowering blood pressure and reducing the risk of related health issues like heart disease and diabetes.

In addition to these physical benefits, exercise offers social opportunities, which are important for emotional health. Group activities like walking clubs, yoga classes, or dance sessions offer a chance to connect with others, fighting the loneliness that some seniors may experience. These social interactions can improve motivation and make exercise more enjoyable, helping seniors stick with their fitness routines.

Safe Exercise Routines to Lower Blood Pressure

When it comes to exercising to lower blood pressure, it's important to choose activities that are safe and appropriate for your fitness level. For seniors, this often means focusing on low-impact exercises that are gentle on the joints while still offering cardiovascular benefits.

Walking is one of the best workouts for seniors. It's easy to do, needs no special equipment, and can be done almost anywhere. Walking at a brisk pace for 30 minutes a day, most days of the week, can greatly lower blood pressure. If 30 minutes seems too long, you can break it into small sessions throughout the day.

Swimming and water exercises are also excellent choices, especially for those with joint pain or arthritis. The water offers resistance, helping to strengthen muscles, while its buoyancy reduces stress on the joints. These exercises offer a full-body workout that improves cardiovascular health and flexibility.

Strength training is another important component of a blood pressure-lowering workout routine. Using light weights, resistance bands, or even body weight exercises like squats and wall push-ups can help build muscle, which in turn can improve metabolism and help keep a healthy weight. Strength training should be done two to three times a week, with a focus on all major muscle parts.

Yoga and Tai Chi are helpful for both physical and mental health. These practices improve flexibility, balance, and strength, while also promoting relaxation and lowering stress—a key factor in managing blood pressure. These exercises can be particularly appealing for seniors as they can be adapted to different fitness levels and done at a pace that feels comfortable.

Before starting any new exercise routine, it's important for seniors to speak with their healthcare provider. They can help determine which activities are safe and suggest modifications to avoid injury. Starting slowly and gradually increasing intensity as fitness improves is a smart method, ensuring that the exercise routine is both effective and sustainable.

Incorporating Activity into Daily Life

Incorporating physical exercise into daily life doesn't have to be daunting. In fact, many simple changes can make a big difference without requiring a structured exercise routine. The goal is to make movement a regular part of your routine, which can help keep blood pressure in check and improve general health.

One of the easiest ways to add more movement to your day is to take the stairs instead of the elevator whenever possible. This small change can strengthen your legs and improve arterial health. If stairs aren't an option, try parking farther away from entrances to increase the number of steps you take each day.

Household chores like gardening, vacuuming, or cleaning can also add to your daily activity level. These tasks keep you moving and can provide a moderate amount of physical exertion that benefits your heart and muscles. Plus, the sense of accomplishment from completing these jobs can boost your mood and overall sense of well-being.

Another way to add more movement is by taking short, frequent breaks during the day to stand up, stretch, and walk around. This is particularly important if you spend a lot of time sitting. Even a few minutes of activity every hour can help improve circulation and reduce the risks linked with prolonged sitting.

Social activities that involve movement, such as dancing, bowling, or even playing with grandchildren, can be both enjoyable and good for your health. These activities don't feel like exercise, but they keep you active and add to your overall fitness. The key is to find things you enjoy so that staying active becomes a natural and enjoyable part of your life.

Overcoming Barriers to Staying Active

While the benefits of physical exercise are clear, many seniors face barriers that make it challenging to stay active. Common obstacles include physical limits, fear of injury, lack of drive, and the misconception that exercise is too difficult or not necessary.

Physical limitations can make some types of exercise difficult or uncomfortable. However, it's important to remember that any movement is better than none, and exercises can be changed to fit individual needs. For example, chair exercises can be an excellent choice for those with limited mobility. These exercises help you to strengthen muscles and improve circulation without putting strain on your joints.

Fear of injury is another common concern, especially for seniors with a history of falls or health issues. To overcome this barrier, focus on low-impact exercises that lower the risk of injury, such as walking, swimming, or gentle yoga.

Starting slowly and using proper techniques can also help avoid injuries. Working with a physical therapist or a fitness instructor who specializes in senior fitness can provide direction and build confidence.

Lack of motivation can be difficult, especially if you're not used to being active. Setting small, achievable goals can help you stay focused. For example, start with a plan to walk for 10 minutes a day, and gradually increase the time as you build stamina. Tracking your progress and celebrating small wins can also keep you motivated.

Finally, some seniors may believe that exercise is too difficult or unnecessary, especially if they've never been very active. It's important to understand that it's never too late to start exercising, and even small increases in activity can have significant health benefits. Education about the benefits of exercise and encouragement from healthcare providers, family, and friends can help change this attitude.

Physical activity is a cornerstone of managing high blood pressure and keeping overall health, especially for seniors. By picking safe exercise routines, incorporating more movement into daily life, and overcoming common barriers, seniors can enjoy the many benefits that regular exercise offers.

These efforts can lead to lower blood pressure, improved physical and mental health, and a better quality of life. Making physical exercise a regular part of your routine is an investment in your health that pays off in countless ways, helping you stay active, independent, and healthy for years to come.

Chapter 9: Weight Management

The Impact of Weight on Blood Pressure

Weight has a significant effect on blood pressure, making it a key factor in managing hypertension, especially for seniors. Carrying excess weight increases the amount of work your heart has to do, as it needs to pump blood through a bigger body mass. This extra work puts additional strain on your arteries, leading to higher blood pressure.

Even a small amount of weight gain can increase blood pressure, which is why maintaining a healthy weight is crucial for those looking to manage or avoid hypertension.

Excess weight, especially around the abdomen, is often associated with an increased risk of high blood pressure. This type of fat, known as visceral fat, surrounds important organs and releases hormones and other substances that can affect blood pressure.

These chemicals can lead to inflammation and insulin resistance, both of which are linked to hypertension. As such, losing even a small amount of weight can have a significant impact on lowering blood pressure and improving overall heart health.

Weight management is not only about reducing the numbers on the scale but also about reducing the risks linked with high blood pressure. By reaching and keeping a healthy weight, you can lower your blood pressure, reduce the strain on your heart, and decrease the chance of complications such as heart disease, stroke, and diabetes. For seniors, managing weight is an important part of keeping independence and overall well-being.

Healthy Weight Loss Strategies for Seniors

Weight loss can be difficult at any age, but it's particularly important to approach it safely and effectively as a senior. The key to healthy weight loss is to focus on gradual changes that promote lasting results rather than quick fixes that can lead to muscle loss, nutrient deficiencies, or other health problems.

One of the most effective methods for healthy weight loss is portion control. As metabolism slows with age, adults often need fewer calories than they did when they were younger. Paying attention to portion sizes and avoiding big meals can help reduce calorie intake without feeling deprived. Using smaller plates, reading food labels, and being aware of serving sizes can all contribute to healthier eating habits.

Balanced, nutrient-dense meals are another cornerstone of good weight loss. The focus should be on consuming a range of fruits, vegetables, lean proteins, whole grains, and healthy fats. These foods provide essential nutrients while making you feel full and satisfied. It's important to avoid empty calories from sugary snacks, processed foods, and high-fat treats that offer little nutritional value.

Regular physical exercise plays a crucial role in weight loss, as it helps burn calories and maintain muscle mass. Incorporating both cardiovascular exercises, like walking or swimming, and strength training exercises can help seniors achieve and keep a healthy weight. Exercise also boosts metabolism and improves overall health, making it easier to manage weight in the long run.

Staying hydrated is another easy yet effective weight loss strategy. Sometimes, thirst is mistaken for hunger, leading to needless snacking. Drinking water throughout the day can help avoid this, reduce calorie intake, and support overall health. Choosing water over sugary drinks also helps cut down on needless calories.

Setting realistic goals is important for lasting weight loss. Seniors should aim for a slow and steady weight loss of about 1 to 2 pounds per week. This pace helps the body to adjust and reduces the risk of muscle loss or other health issues. It's also important to celebrate small victories along the way, which can help keep motivation and encourage long-term success.

Finally, seeking help can make a big difference in achieving weight loss goals. This might involve working with a healthcare provider, a chef, or joining a weight loss group. Having a support system can provide accountability, encouragement, and practical help tailored to individual needs.

Maintaining a Healthy Weight Long-Term

Maintaining a healthy weight over the long term takes ongoing effort and lifestyle changes that become part of your daily routine. For seniors, the focus should be on building habits that are sustainable, enjoyable, and supportive of overall health.

One of the most important aspects of keeping a healthy weight is continuing with regular physical activity. Exercise not only helps keep the weight off but also offers numerous health benefits, including improved cardiovascular health, better balance and rhythm, and enhanced mental well-being. Finding things that you enjoy, such as walking, dancing, or gardening, makes it easier to stay active and keep the weight off.

Consistent, thoughtful eating is also key to long-term weight maintenance. This means being aware of what and how much you're eating, even after you've hit your weight loss goals. Continue to focus on portion control, healthy meals, and avoiding processed foods. It's also important to pay attention to hunger and fullness cues, eating when you're hungry and stopping when you're filled.

Regular self-monitoring can help you stay on track with your weight control goals. This might include weighing yourself weekly, keeping a food log, or tracking your activity levels. Monitoring your progress can help you catch any small changes before they become bigger problems, allowing you to make adjustments as needed.

Planning for challenges is another important part of keeping a healthy weight. Life events, worry, or changes in routine can sometimes lead to weight gain. Being prepared with strategies to handle these situations—such as having healthy snacks on hand, sticking to a regular exercise plan, or practicing stress-relief techniques—can help you stay on track.

Staying linked to a support system can also be crucial for long-term success. Whether it's friends, family, or a health worker, having people who encourage and support your healthy lifestyle can make a big difference in maintaining your weight. Regular check-ins, whether in person or online, can provide motivation and accountability.

Lastly, maintaining a positive attitude is important. Weight control is a lifelong journey, and it's normal to experience ups and downs along the way. It's important to focus on the progress you've made, rather than any setbacks, and to keep in mind the overall benefits of keeping a healthy weight—such as feeling better, having more energy, and reducing your risk of chronic diseases.

Managing weight successfully is a key component of controlling blood pressure, especially for seniors. By understanding the effect of weight on blood pressure, adopting healthy weight loss strategies, and committing to keeping a healthy weight long-term, seniors can significantly improve their overall health and quality of life. These efforts not only help lower blood pressure but also reduce the chance of related health issues, leading to a healthier, more fulfilling life.

Chapter 10: Stress Management

Understanding the Stress-Pressure Connection

Stress is an inevitable part of life, and while it can sometimes be a positive force that motivates us to take action, chronic stress is a major contributor to high blood pressure (hypertension). Understanding the link between stress and blood pressure is crucial for managing hypertension, especially for seniors who may face unique stressors related to aging, health, and lifestyle changes.

When you face a stressful situation, your body undergoes a series of physiological changes known as the "fight-or-flight" response. This response is meant to help you deal with immediate threats by preparing your body for quick action. During this response, your body releases stress hormones like adrenaline and cortisol, which briefly increase your heart rate and constrict your blood vessels. This leads to a rise in blood pressure, ensuring that enough blood and oxygen reach your muscles and organs to handle the perceived danger.

While this temporary spike in blood pressure is normal and normally subsides once the stressful situation is over, chronic stress can lead to sustained high blood pressure.

When stress becomes a constant part of your life, your body stays in a heightened state of alertness, with elevated levels of stress hormones and persistent increases in blood pressure. Over time, this can cause long-term damage to your cardiovascular system, raising the risk of heart disease, stroke, and other serious health conditions.

For example, picture a scenario where you're constantly worried about finances, health issues, or family problems. This ongoing stress keeps your body in a state of heightened arousal, causing your blood vessels to stay constricted and your heart to work harder than usual. If this situation continues without effective stress management, it can lead to chronic hypertension, putting you at greater risk for cardiovascular problems.

Techniques for Reducing Stress: Meditation, Yoga, and Relaxation Exercises

Given the strong connection between stress and high blood pressure, learning how to manage stress effectively is important for maintaining heart health. There are several proven methods that can help reduce stress and, by extension, lower blood pressure. Among the most beneficial are meditation, yoga, and relaxation exercises.

1. Meditation:

Meditation is a practice that involves focusing the mind on a particular object, thought, or action to achieve a mentally clear and emotionally calm state. There are different types of meditation, but they all share a common goal: reducing stress by calming the mind and relaxing the body.

One of the most famous forms of meditation is mindfulness meditation, which involves paying attention to the present moment without judgment. During mindfulness meditation, you focus on your breath, bodily feelings, or a specific thought, gently bringing your attention back whenever your mind wanders. This practice helps to reduce stress by promoting relaxation and reducing the body's stress reaction.

Research has shown that regular meditation can lower blood pressure by reducing the activity of the sympathetic nervous system (which controls the fight-or-flight reaction) and enhancing the parasympathetic nervous system (which promotes relaxation). For example, a study released in the Journal of Hypertension found that participants who practiced meditation regularly experienced significant reductions in both systolic and diastolic blood pressure.

2. Yoga:

Yoga is a mind-body practice that combines physical postures, breathing exercises, and meditation to promote general well-being. It has been practiced for thousands of years and is known for its ability to reduce stress, improve flexibility, and increase mental clarity.

Yoga is particularly effective for reducing stress because it promotes mindfulness, deep breathing, and physical relaxation. The mixture of these elements helps to calm the mind, reduce the release of stress hormones, and lower blood pressure. Certain yoga poses, such as forward bends, twists, and inversions, are especially helpful for relieving tension and promoting relaxation.

For instance, the "Child's Pose" (Balasana) is a simple yet effective yoga pose that helps to release tension in the back, shoulders, and neck while promoting deep, calming breaths. Similarly, the "Legs-Up-the-Wall Pose" (Viparita Karani) is an inversion pose that pushes blood flow away from the legs and toward the heart, helping to lower blood pressure and reduce stress.

3. Relaxation Exercises:

Relaxation techniques, such as deep breathing, progressive muscle relaxation, and guided imagery, are powerful tools for managing stress and lowering blood pressure. These techniques work by slowing down the body's stress reaction and promoting a state of calm and relaxation.

● Deep Breathing: This method involves taking slow, deep breaths to activate the body's relaxation response. By focusing on your breath and breathing deeply from the diaphragm, you can lower your heart rate, reduce stress, and lower blood pressure. An effective deep breathing exercise is the 4-7-8 technique: inhale deeply through your nose for a count of four, hold your breath for a count of seven, and release slowly through your mouth for a count of eight.

● Progressive Muscle Relaxation (PMR): PMR is a method that involves tensing and then slowly relaxing each muscle group in the body. This method helps to release physical tension and promotes a feeling of calm. To practice PMR, start with your toes and work your way up to your head, tensing each muscle group for a few seconds before slowly relaxing the tension. This exercise not only relaxes your muscles but also calms your mind, lowering stress and blood pressure.

●   Guided Imagery: This relaxation technique involves visualizing calming and peaceful images or situations to reduce stress. By engaging your imagination and focusing on a serene environment—such as a beach, forest, or mountain—you can distract your mind from stressors and induce a state of relaxation. Guided imagery can be practiced with the help of recorded audio sessions or simply by making your own mental imagery.

Developing a Stress-Reduction Plan

Effectively managing stress requires a thoughtful and personalized approach. Developing a stress-reduction plan tailored to your needs and lifestyle can help you consistently apply stress management techniques and keep a healthy blood pressure. Here's how to build a practical and effective stress-reduction plan:

1. Identify Your Stress Triggers:

The first step in creating a stress-reduction plan is identifying the specific situations, activities, or thoughts that trigger your stress. These triggers can vary widely from person to person and may include work-related pressures, health issues, cash worries, or interpersonal conflicts. By recognizing what causes you stress, you can take specific steps to address or mitigate these triggers.

For example, if financial concerns are a major source of stress, you might benefit from creating a budget, getting financial advice, or finding ways to increase your income. If health problems are a trigger, focusing on lifestyle changes, regular exercise, and medical consultations can help you regain control and reduce stress.

2. Incorporate Stress-Reduction Techniques into Your Daily Routine:

Once you've identified your stress triggers, the next step is to incorporate stress-reduction methods into your daily routine. Consistency is key when it comes to managing stress, so it's important to make these routines a regular part of your life.

- Morning Routine: Start your day with a few minutes of meditation or deep breathing techniques. This can help set a positive tone for the day and give you the resilience to handle stressors as they arise.

● Midday Breaks: If possible, add yoga or relaxation exercises into your midday routine. Even a short walk, paired with mindful breathing, can help break the cycle of stress and refresh your mind.

● Evening Wind-Down: Use the evening to practice progressive muscle relaxation or guided images. These methods can help you unwind after a long day, reduce any accumulated stress, and prepare your body for restful sleep.

3. Set Realistic Goals and Expectations:

Stress often comes from setting unrealistic goals or having expectations that are too high. To reduce stress, it's important to set realistic goals and be kind to yourself when things don't go as planned. Break larger jobs into smaller, manageable steps and celebrate your progress along the way.

For instance, if you're working on a long-term project, set daily or weekly milestones rather than focusing solely on the end goal. This method can help reduce the pressure you place on yourself and make the process more enjoyable and less stressful.

4. Build a Support System:

Having a strong support system is important for managing stress effectively. Surround yourself with friends, family, or workers who can offer encouragement, advice, and a listening ear when you need it. Don't hesitate to reach out to others for help, whether it's for physical assistance or emotional support.

Additionally, consider joining a support group or getting professional counseling if you're dealing with chronic stress or specific life challenges. Talking to others who are going through similar experiences can provide comfort and new views on managing stress.

5. Practice Self-Care and Healthy Habits:

Self-care is a crucial component of any stress-reduction plan. Make time for things that you enjoy and that bring you peace, whether it's reading, gardening, listening to music, or spending time in nature. Regular physical exercise, a balanced diet, and sufficient sleep are also important for maintaining your overall well-being and reducing stress.

For example, if you love being outdoors, consider scheduling regular walks in the park or time spent gardening. These hobbies not only provide physical exercise but also offer a mental break from daily stressors.

6. Monitor Your Progress and Adjust as Needed:

Finally, it's important to regularly check your progress and adjust your stress-reduction plan as needed. Pay attention to how your body and mind respond to the methods you're using. If something isn't going as well as you'd hoped, don't be afraid to try different approaches or seek additional support.

Keep track of your stress levels and blood pressure readings over time to see how your efforts are impacting your general health. This data can provide useful insights and motivation to continue your stress-management practices.

Managing stress is a vital aspect of keeping healthy blood pressure, especially for seniors who may face unique challenges related to aging and lifestyle changes. By understanding the link between stress and blood pressure and incorporating

Chapter 11: Sleep and Blood Pressure

The Importance of Quality Sleep

Sleep is a fundamental part of our health, having a crucial role in maintaining various bodily functions, including the regulation of blood pressure. Quality sleep allows the body to rest, repair, and rejuvenate, which is especially important for heart health. When you sleep, your blood pressure automatically dips, giving your heart and blood vessels a much-needed break. This nocturnal drop in blood pressure is known as "nocturnal dipping," and it's important for cardiovascular health.

Consistently getting enough quality sleep helps keep this healthy blood pressure pattern. In contrast, poor sleep, whether due to insufficient length or poor quality, can disrupt this natural dip, leading to higher blood pressure levels throughout the day. Over time, chronic sleep deprivation or consistently poor sleep can lead to sustained high blood pressure, also known as hypertension.

For example, a person who regularly sleeps for only five or six hours a night may not experience the full benefits of nighttime dipping. This lack of rest can prevent the heart from fully recovering, causing a strain that leads to higher blood pressure during waking hours. As a result, the risk of getting hypertension rises, along with the potential for more serious cardiovascular conditions such as heart disease and stroke.

Furthermore, quality sleep affects the body's ability to handle stress, which is another key factor in blood pressure regulation. During deep sleep stages, the brain processes stress and emotions, helping to stabilize mood and reduce the physiological stress reaction that can elevate blood pressure. Without adequate deep sleep, the body's stress response may stay heightened, leading to persistent elevations in blood pressure.

Sleep Disorders and Their Impact on Blood Pressure

Sleep disorders are common among seniors and can have a significant effect on blood pressure. Conditions like sleep apnea, insomnia, and restless legs syndrome not only disrupt sleep but also directly add to the development and worsening of hypertension.

1. Sleep Apnea:

Sleep apnea is a sleep disorder marked by repeated interruptions in breathing during sleep. These pauses, known as apneas, can last from a few seconds to a minute and can occur dozens of times per hour. The most common type is obstructive sleep apnea (OSA), where the airway becomes partly or fully blocked during sleep, leading to reduced oxygen levels in the blood.

When breathing is interrupted, the body reacts by quickly waking up to restore normal breathing. This constant cycle of waking and sleeping puts a strain on the cardiovascular system, causing blood pressure to spike each time the body responds to a lack of oxygen. Over time, these repeated spikes can lead to continued high blood pressure.

Moreover, sleep apnea is often linked with other cardiovascular risks, such as atrial fibrillation and heart failure. Studies have shown that untreated sleep apnea significantly increases the chance of developing hypertension and can make existing high blood pressure more difficult to control. For example, a person with untreated sleep apnea may experience persistent hypertension despite taking medication, simply because the underlying sleep disorder is not being handled.

2. Insomnia:

Insomnia, the inability to fall asleep or stay asleep, is another common sleep problem that can negatively affect blood pressure. Chronic insomnia leads to a reduction in the overall quality and amount of sleep, which can disrupt the natural regulation of blood pressure.

When a person has insomnia, they may experience increased amounts of stress and anxiety, both of which can raise blood pressure. Additionally, the lack of restful sleep can lead to a hyperactive sympathetic nervous system, which controls the body's "fight-or-flight" reaction. This heightened state of arousal can cause the heart to work harder and blood vessels to tighten, resulting in elevated blood pressure.

Over time, chronic insomnia can add to the development of hypertension and increase the risk of heart disease. For example, a person who struggles with insomnia may find themselves feeling constantly fatigued and stressed, which can lead to unhealthy coping strategies such as poor dietary choices or lack of exercise, further exacerbating the risk of high blood pressure.

3. Restless Legs Syndrome (RLS):

Restless Legs Syndrome is a neurological problem that causes an irresistible urge to move the legs, usually followed by uncomfortable sensations such as tingling, aching, or itching. These sensations typically increase at night, making it difficult to fall asleep or stay asleep.

The frequent movement and discomfort caused by RLS can lead to fragmented sleep, preventing the body from entering the deep sleep stages that are important for blood pressure regulation. As a result, people with RLS may experience higher blood pressure levels, both at night and during the day.

Moreover, the chronic sleep deprivation associated with RLS can lead to increased worry and fatigue, both of which can further elevate blood pressure. Managing RLS is important not only for better sleep quality but also for protecting cardiovascular health.

Tips for Better Sleep

Improving sleep quality is important for maintaining healthy blood pressure levels. Here are some useful tips to help you achieve better sleep:

1. Establish a Consistent Sleep Schedule:

Going to bed and getting up at the same time every day, even on weekends, helps regulate your body's internal clock. This consistency makes it easier to fall asleep at night and wake up feeling refreshed in the morning. A regular sleep schedule also promotes the natural nocturnal dipping of blood pressure, which is good for heart health.

For example, if you aim to get seven to eight hours of sleep, try making a bedtime of 10:00 p.m. and waking up at 6:00 a.m. each day. Over time, your body will adjust to this habit, making it easier to fall asleep and wake up without an alarm.

2. Create a Relaxing Bedtime Routine:

Establishing a calming pre-sleep practice can signal to your body that it's time to wind down. Activities such as reading a book, taking a warm bath, or performing relaxation exercises like deep breathing or meditation can help prepare your mind and body for sleep.

Avoid stimulating activities before bed, such as watching television, using electronic devices, or participating in intense discussions. The blue light emitted by screens can interfere with the production of melatonin, the hormone that controls sleep, making it harder to fall asleep.

3. Optimize Your Sleep Environment:

Your sleep environment plays a significant part in the quality of your sleep. Ensure that your bedroom is cool, quiet, and dark, as these conditions are beneficial to better sleep. Consider using blackout shades, earplugs, or a white noise machine if necessary.

Investing in a nice mattress and pillows that support your body can also make a difference in how well you sleep. A supportive mattress can alleviate pressure points and reduce the chance of waking up with aches and pains.

4. Be Mindful of Your Diet and Hydration:

What you eat and drink before bed can impact your sleep. Avoid large meals, caffeine, and booze in the hours leading up to bedtime, as these can disrupt sleep. Caffeine is a stimulant that can keep you awake, while booze may cause fragmented sleep later in the night.

However, it's also important to stay refreshed. Dehydration can cause pain and restlessness, making it harder to sleep. Aim to drink enough water throughout the day, but try to limit fluids in the evening to reduce the chance of waking up to use the bathroom.

5. Manage Stress and Anxiety:

Stress and anxiety are regular causes of sleep disturbances. Incorporating stress management methods into your daily routine can help calm your mind and improve your sleep quality.

Practices such as mindfulness meditation, deep breathing exercises, and gentle yoga can help lower stress and promote relaxation before bed.

If your mind tends to race with worries as soon as you lie down, try keeping a journal by your bedside. Writing down your thoughts and worries before bed can help clear your mind and make it easier to fall asleep.

6. Get Regular Exercise:

Regular physical exercise can improve sleep quality by reducing stress and tiring the body, making it easier to fall asleep. However, try to avoid intense exercise close to bedtime, as it can be stimulating and interfere with your ability to fall asleep.

Aim for at least 30 minutes of moderate exercise, such as walking, swimming, or riding, most days of the week. Exercise not only helps better sleep but also has the added benefit of lowering blood pressure.

7. Seek Help for Sleep Disorders:

If you think you have a sleep disorder such as sleep apnea, insomnia, or restless legs syndrome, it's important to seek help from a healthcare professional. Proper diagnosis and treatment can greatly improve your sleep quality and help manage your blood pressure.

For example, if you have sleep apnea, your doctor may suggest a Continuous Positive Airway Pressure (CPAP) machine, which helps keep your airway open during sleep. Treating sleep apnea can reduce blood pressure and lower the chance of cardiovascular complications.

Quality sleep is essential for maintaining healthy blood pressure levels, especially as we age. By understanding the importance of sleep, recognizing the effect of sleep disorders, and adopting strategies for better sleep, you can take significant steps toward improving your overall health and lowering the risk of hypertension. Prioritizing sleep is a vital part of managing blood pressure and safeguarding your heart for the long run.

Chapter 12: Avoiding Tobacco and Limiting Alcohol

How Smoking Affects Blood Pressure

Smoking is one of the most important risk factors for the development of high blood pressure and other cardiovascular diseases. The harmful effects of smoking on blood pressure are both instant and long-term.

When you smoke a cigarette, the nicotine in tobacco causes a quick increase in blood pressure and heart rate. This happens because nicotine stimulates the adrenal glands to release adrenaline, a hormone that constricts blood vessels and pushes the heart to beat faster. This constriction of blood vessels increases the difficulty against which the heart has to pump blood, leading to elevated blood pressure.

Moreover, the carbon monoxide in cigarette smoke lowers the amount of oxygen that your blood can carry. This means your heart has to work harder to give enough oxygen to your body's tissues, further increasing blood pressure. Over time, smoking damages the lining of the arteries, making them more prone to atherosclerosis, a disease where fatty deposits build up on the artery walls.

Atherosclerosis narrows the vessels and increases blood pressure even more. This chronic elevation in blood pressure due to smoking significantly increases the risk of heart disease, stroke, and other major health problems.

For instance, a long-term smoker is at a much higher chance of developing chronic hypertension (high blood pressure) compared to a non-smoker. The continuous exposure to nicotine and other harmful chemicals in tobacco smoke keeps the blood vessels in a state of constant tension and inflammation, leading to continued high blood pressure.

Strategies for Quitting Smoking

Quitting smoking is one of the most effective ways to lower blood pressure and reduce the chance of cardiovascular disease. However, quitting can be difficult due to nicotine's addictive nature. Here are some techniques that can help you quit smoking successfully:

1. Set a Quit Date:

Choosing a set date to quit smoking can help you mentally prepare for the change. Make this day important, perhaps by choosing a birthday, anniversary, or a date that has personal meaning. Once you've set your quit date, prepare by slightly reducing the number of cigarettes you smoke each day. This can help ease the transition and lessen withdrawal symptoms.

2. Identify Triggers and Avoid Them:

Understanding what triggers your urge to smoke is important. Common triggers include stress, social settings, drinking alcohol, or even certain times of day. Once you identify these triggers, you can create strategies to avoid or cope with them. For example, if you usually smoke while drinking coffee, try switching to tea or going for a walk instead. If stress is a major trigger, practice relaxation methods like deep breathing, meditation, or yoga.

3. Use Nicotine Replacement Therapy (NRT):

Nicotine replacement therapy (NRT) can help reduce withdrawal symptoms by giving a small, controlled amount of nicotine without the harmful chemicals found in cigarettes. NRT products come in different forms, including patches, gum, lozenges, inhalers, and nasal sprays. These products can help you gently wean off nicotine while minimizing cravings and withdrawal symptoms.

For instance, starting with a nicotine patch can provide a steady release of nicotine throughout the day, reducing the desire to smoke. As your body changes, you can gradually lower the dose until you no longer need the patch.

4. Consider Prescription Medications:

There are prescription medications available that can help you stop smoking by reducing cravings and withdrawal symptoms. Two widely prescribed medications are varenicline (Chantix) and bupropion (Zyban). Varenicline works by blocking the effects of nicotine on the brain, making smoking less enjoyable, while bupropion is an antidepressant that can help lessen cravings and withdrawal symptoms.

These medications are usually prescribed for a limited time and should be taken under the direction of a healthcare provider. They can be particularly helpful for people who have tried to quit smoking multiple times without success.

5. Seek Support:

Quitting smoking is easier when you have help. Tell your family, friends, and co-workers about your plan to quit so they can offer support and help you stay on track. You might also consider joining a support group or participating in a smoking quit program, either in person or online. These programs provide tools, counseling, and support from others who are also trying to quit.

For example, many communities offer free smoking cessation classes or support groups, where you can share your experiences and challenges with others who are on the same road.

6. Stay Positive and Persistent:

Quitting smoking is a process that often involves hurdles. If you slip up and smoke a cigarette, don't be too hard on yourself. Instead, view it as a learning experience and recommit to your goal of stopping. Staying upbeat and persistent is key to long-term success. Remind yourself of the health benefits of quitting, such as lower blood pressure, reduced risk of heart disease, and better lung function.

Alcohol Consumption: What's Safe and What's Not

Alcohol consumption can have a complex link with blood pressure. While moderate alcohol consumption may have some cardiovascular benefits, excessive drinking is a well-known risk factor for high blood pressure and other health problems.

1. Understanding Moderate Drinking:

Moderate alcohol consumption is usually defined as up to one drink per day for women and up to two drinks per day for men. One drink is usually considered to be:

- 12 ounces of beer - 5 ounces of wine
- 1.5 ounces of distilled drinks (like vodka, whiskey, or rum)

Moderate drinking may have some heart benefits, such as raising "good" HDL cholesterol levels, but these benefits must be weighed against the risks, especially for those with high blood pressure or a history of hypertension.

2. The Dangers of Excessive Drinking:

Excessive alcohol intake is harmful to your health and can lead to a number of serious issues, including high blood pressure. Heavy drinking, defined as consuming more than three drinks in one sitting or drinking heavily over time, can cause a large and sustained increase in blood pressure.

Alcohol raises blood pressure by several processes, including stimulating the sympathetic nervous system, which controls the body's "fight or flight" response. This excitement can lead to vasoconstriction (narrowing of blood vessels), which increases blood pressure. Over time, heavy alcohol use can lead to chronic hypertension and an increased chance of heart disease, stroke, and other cardiovascular problems.

For example, someone who frequently consumes alcohol in large quantities may experience spikes in blood pressure that, over time, lead to the development of chronic hypertension. This risk is particularly high for people who drink heavily and have other risk factors for high blood pressure, such as obesity or a family history of hypertension.

3. Tips for Safe Alcohol Consumption:

To manage blood pressure properly, it's important to limit alcohol consumption. Here are some tips for drinking safely:

- Stick to Moderation: If you choose to drink, do so in moderation. Keeping your alcohol intake within the recommended limits can help avoid alcohol-related increases in blood pressure.

- measure Your Blood Pressure: If you drink alcohol, it's important to measure your blood pressure regularly. Some people are more sensitive to the blood pressure-raising effects of alcohol than others. If you find that your blood pressure rises after drinking, consider reducing or eliminating alcohol from your diet.

- Avoid Binge Drinking: Binge drinking, or taking a large amount of alcohol in a short period of time, can cause a sudden spike in blood pressure. Avoid this drinking habit to protect your cardiovascular health.

- Choose Low-Sodium Mixers: If you enjoy mixed drinks, opt for low-sodium mixers like club soda, tonic water, or freshly squeezed fruit juice. High-sodium mixers, such as many canned or bottled sodas, can add to increased blood pressure.

- Stay Hydrated: Alcohol can lead to dehydration, which can affect blood pressure. Drinking water between alcoholic drinks can help you stay hydrated and reduce the amount of alcohol you consume overall.

- Be Mindful of Your Triggers: Just as with smoking, certain social settings or stressors may prompt you to drink more. Be aware of these triggers and have a plan in place to handle them without relying on alcohol.

Avoiding tobacco and limiting alcohol consumption are critical steps in managing blood pressure and lowering the risk of cardiovascular disease. Smoking has a direct and harmful effect on blood pressure, while excessive alcohol intake can contribute to the development of hypertension. By quitting smoking and drinking alcohol in moderation, you can greatly improve your heart health and overall well-being. Taking these steps not only lowers your blood pressure but also improves your quality of life, helping you live a longer, healthier life.

Chapter 13: Medications for High Blood Pressure

Overview of Common Blood Pressure Medications

High blood pressure, or hypertension, is a common disease, especially among seniors. Managing it often requires a mix of lifestyle changes and medications. There are several types of medicines available to help control blood pressure, each working in different ways to lower it and reduce the risk of heart disease, stroke, and other complications. Here's an overview of the most popular classes of blood pressure medications:

1. Diuretics (Water Pills): Diuretics are often the first type of medication given for high blood pressure. They help your kidneys clear excess sodium (salt) and water from your body, which reduces blood volume and, in turn, lowers blood pressure. Common diuretics include hydrochlorothiazide, chlorthalidone, and furosemide. Diuretics are especially helpful for older adults and those with heart failure.

2. ACE Inhibitors (Angiotensin-Converting Enzyme Inhibitors): ACE inhibitors help relax blood vessels by preventing the formation of a hormone called angiotensin II, which usually causes blood vessels to narrow. By stopping this hormone, ACE inhibitors make it easier for your heart to pump blood. Common ACE inhibitors include lisinopril, enalapril, and ramipril. They are particularly helpful for people with diabetes or chronic kidney disease.

3. ARBs (Angiotensin II Receptor Blockers): ARBs work similarly to ACE inhibitors but stop the action of angiotensin II directly on the blood vessels. This also helps to soften and widen blood vessels. Common ARBs include losartan, valsartan, and irbesartan. ARBs are often used in people who experience side effects like a chronic cough from ACE inhibitors.

4. Calcium Channel Blockers: These medications keep calcium from entering the cells of your heart and blood vessel walls, resulting in lower blood pressure. Calcium channel blockers can also help slow your heart rate, which lowers the heart's workload. Common examples include amlodipine, diltiazem, and verapamil. These drugs are particularly helpful for older adults and those with certain heart conditions.

5. Beta-Blockers: Beta-blockers work by blocking the effects of adrenaline on your heart. This slows down your heart rate and lowers the force of your heartbeats, lowering blood pressure. Common beta-blockers include metoprolol, atenolol, and propranolol. These medications are often given to people who have heart conditions such as angina or a history of heart attacks.

6. Alpha-Blockers: Alpha-blockers lower blood pressure by blocking nerve signals that cause blood vessels to tighten. This helps blood to flow more freely through the vessels. Common alpha-blockers include doxazosin and prazosin. They are sometimes used in combination with other blood pressure medicines.

7. Vasodilators: Vasodilators directly relax the muscles in the walls of your blood vessels, causing the vessels to widen and blood pressure to drop. Hydralazine and minoxidil are examples of vasodilators. These medications are usually reserved for cases where other blood pressure medications are not helpful enough.

How These Medications Work

Each type of blood pressure medicine works differently to help lower blood pressure:

- Diuretics reduce the volume of blood by eliminating extra water and salt through urination, which lowers the pressure on your artery walls.
- ACE Inhibitors and ARBs target the renin-angiotensin system, a hormone system that controls blood pressure. By

interfering with this system, these drugs keep blood vessels from narrowing, which helps to lower blood pressure.

- Calcium Channel Blockers prevent calcium from entering heart and blood vessel cells, which relaxes the blood vessels and lowers heart rate and blood pressure.
- Beta-Blockers lower the workload on your heart by slowing your heart rate and decreasing the force of your heart's contractions.
- Alpha-Blockers and Vasodilators directly relax blood vessels, making it easier for blood to flow through them, thereby lowering blood pressure.

These medications can be given alone or in combination, depending on the severity of your hypertension and any other health conditions you might have.

Potential Side Effects and How to Manage Them

While blood pressure medications are helpful, they can also cause side effects. Understanding these potential side effects and how to handle them can help you stick with your treatment plan.

1. Diuretics:

Side Effects: Diuretics can cause greater urination, which may lead to dehydration and electrolyte imbalances. They may also cause dizziness, tiredness, or muscle cramps.

Management: To avoid dehydration, make sure you drink plenty of water. Your doctor may also monitor your potassium levels and suggest potassium-rich foods or supplements if needed.

2. ACE Inhibitors:

Side Effects: Common side effects include a prolonged dry cough, elevated blood potassium levels, and dizziness, especially after the first dose.

Management: If the cough becomes annoying, your doctor might switch you to an ARB, which usually does not cause this side effect. Regular blood tests can help check potassium levels.

3. ARBs:

Side Effects: Similar to ACE inhibitors, ARBs can cause dizziness and elevated blood potassium levels but are less likely to cause a chronic cough.

Management: As with ACE inhibitors, your doctor will watch your potassium levels and may adjust your diet or medications accordingly.

4. Calcium Channel Blockers:

Side Effects: These can include swelling in the legs or feet, dizziness, and headaches.

Management: Elevating your legs can help reduce swelling, and taking your medicine with food might lessen headaches. If side effects continue, your doctor may adjust the dosage.

5. Beta-Blockers:

Side Effects: Possible side effects include fatigue, cold hands and feet, slow heart rate, and sadness.

Management: To manage fatigue, try to balance rest with gentle physical exercise. If you experience a slow heart rate or severe coldness in your extremities, call your doctor. Adjustments to your medicine might be necessary.

6. Alpha-Blockers:

Side Effects: These include dizziness or fainting, especially after the first dose, and a fast heart rate.

Management: Take your first dose at bedtime to lower the risk of dizziness. If you continue to feel dizzy, your doctor may change your dosage.

7. Vasodilators:

Side Effects: Vasodilators can cause headaches, rapid heartbeat, and fluid buildup.

Management: Your doctor may prescribe a diuretic to manage fluid retention or change your dosage to minimize side effects.

Tips for Medication Adherence

Taking your blood pressure medication as prescribed is important for effectively managing hypertension. However, it's not uncommon to forget doses or stop taking medicine due to side effects or feeling better. Here are some tips to help you stick to your medicine regimen:

1. Establish a Routine: Take your medicine at the same time each day. Pairing it with a daily habit, like brushing your teeth or having breakfast, can help you remember.

2. Use a Pill Organizer: A pill organizer can help you keep track of your medications and ensure you're taking the right amount at the right time. Weekly or monthly organizers are available, based on your preference.

3. Set Reminders: Use alarms on your phone or a medication reminder app to tell you when it's time to take your medication. Some apps also allow you to track your medication usage and share the information with your healthcare provider.

4. Simplify Your Medication Regimen: If you're taking multiple drugs, ask your doctor if it's possible to simplify your regimen. Sometimes, combination pills that contain more than one type of medication can lower the number of pills you need to take each day.

5. Keep a Medication Journal: Documenting how you feel after taking your medication, any side effects you experience, and any missed doses can help you and your doctor spot patterns and make adjustments as needed.

6. Communicate with Your Healthcare Provider: If you're suffering side effects or having trouble adhering to your medication regimen, don't hesitate to talk to your doctor. They can change your dosage or switch you to a different medication to better suit your needs.

7. Stay Informed: Understanding the importance of your medicine and how it works can encourage you to take it consistently. If you have questions about your medicine, ask your doctor or pharmacist for more information.

Medications are an important part of managing high blood pressure, especially when lifestyle changes alone are not enough. Understanding how these medications work, being aware of possible side effects, and following tips for adherence can help you successfully manage your blood pressure and reduce the risk of serious health complications.

Chapter 14: Alternative and Complementary Therapies

Herbal Supplements and Natural Remedies

In recent years, there has been greater interest in using herbal supplements and natural remedies as alternatives or complements to conventional high blood pressure treatments. Many people are drawn to these choices because they are perceived as more "natural" and, in some cases, may have fewer side effects than prescription medications. However, while some herbal supplements and natural remedies can help control blood pressure, it's important to approach them with caution and consult your healthcare provider before incorporating them into your routine.

Common Herbal Supplements for Blood Pressure

1. Garlic:

Garlic is one of the most well-known natural treatments for lowering blood pressure. Studies have shown that garlic can help relax blood vessels and lower systolic and diastolic blood pressure. This effect is credited to allicin, a compound released when garlic is crushed or chopped. Garlic supplements are available in different forms, including tablets, capsules, and aged garlic extract.

2. Hawthorn:

Hawthorn has been used in traditional medicine for ages to treat heart-related conditions. It is thought to improve blood flow, reduce blood pressure, and strengthen the heart muscle. Hawthorn is usually taken as a supplement in the form of capsules, tablets, or liquid extracts.

3. Omega-3 Fatty Acids:

Found in fish oil and flaxseed oil, omega-3 fatty acids are well-known for their heart health benefits. They help lower blood pressure by reducing inflammation, improving blood vessel function, and lowering blood clotting. Omega-3 supplements are typically available as fish oil capsules or flaxseed oil.

4. Coenzyme Q10 (CoQ10):

CoQ10 is a naturally occurring antioxidant that plays a key role in energy production within cells.

Some studies suggest that CoQ10 supplements can help lower blood pressure, especially in people with hypertension. It is available in different forms, including soft gels and tablets.

5. L-Arginine:

L-arginine is an amino acid that the body uses to make nitric oxide, a compound that relaxes blood vessels and lowers blood pressure. Some research has shown that L-arginine supplements may help reduce blood pressure, especially in people with mild hypertension.

The Role of Diet in Natural Blood Pressure Management

In addition to herbal supplements, dietary choices can greatly affect blood pressure. The DASH (Dietary Approaches to Stop Hypertension) diet, which emphasizes fruits, vegetables, whole grains, and low-fat dairy products, is a well-established dietary method to lower blood pressure. Incorporating potassium-rich foods like bananas, spinach, and sweet potatoes, as well as reducing sodium intake, can further improve the blood pressure-lowering effects of your diet.

The Role of Acupuncture, Massage, and Other Therapies

Beyond herbal supplements and dietary changes, several alternative therapies are widely used to help manage high blood pressure. These therapies often focus on reducing stress and boosting relaxation, which can positively impact blood pressure levels.

Acupuncture

Acupuncture, a key component of traditional Chinese medicine, involves inserting thin needles into specific points on the body to stimulate energy flow and balance bodily processes. Some studies show that acupuncture may help lower blood pressure by promoting relaxation and reducing stress. It is thought to affect the autonomic nervous system, which controls blood pressure, heart rate, and other involuntary functions.

While acupuncture can be a useful complementary therapy, it is usually not recommended as a sole treatment for high blood pressure. Combining acupuncture with conventional treatments like medicine and lifestyle changes may offer the best results. As with any therapy, it's important to seek a qualified and licensed acupuncturist to ensure safe and effective care.

Massage Therapy

Massage therapy is another alternative treatment that can help lower blood pressure by reducing stress and boosting relaxation. Regular massage sessions have been shown to reduce systolic and diastolic blood pressure, likely due to the reduction of stress hormones like cortisol and the improvement of blood circulation.

Different types of massage, such as Swedish, deep tissue, and aromatherapy massage, can be tailored to individual tastes and needs. However, it's important to communicate with your massage therapist about your condition, as certain techniques may need to be modified for people with hypertension.

Mind-Body Practices: Yoga and Meditation

Mind-body practices such as yoga and meditation are generally recognized for their ability to reduce stress and improve overall well-being. These practices can be particularly helpful for managing high blood pressure, as stress is a known contributor to hypertension.

Yoga:

Yoga combines physical postures, breathing exercises, and meditation to encourage relaxation and lower stress. Studies have shown that regular yoga practice can lower blood pressure, improve heart rate variability, and enhance general cardiovascular health. Specific yoga poses, such as forward bends and restorative poses, are thought to have a calming effect on the nervous system, which can help lower blood pressure.

Meditation: Meditation includes focusing the mind and eliminating distractions to achieve a state of deep relaxation and mental clarity.

Mindfulness meditation, in particular, has been shown to lower blood pressure by promoting relaxation and reducing stress levels. Practicing meditation for as little as 10-15 minutes a day can have a positive effect on blood pressure and general health.

Evaluating the Safety and Effectiveness of Alternative Treatments

While alternative and complementary therapies can offer benefits for handling high blood pressure, it's crucial to approach them with an informed and cautious mindset. Not all alternative treatments are safe or successful, and some may interact with prescription medications or worsen certain health conditions. Here are some important factors when evaluating alternative treatments:

Consult Your Healthcare Provider

Before starting any alternative or complementary therapy, it's important to consult your healthcare provider. They can help you understand the possible risks and benefits of the therapy, as well as how it might interact with your current treatment plan. For example, some herbal supplements can interact with blood pressure medications or cause unwanted side effects.

Research and Evidence

Not all alternative therapies have been fully studied or proven effective in clinical trials. When considering a new treatment, it's important to research the available evidence and look for studies that support its safety and success. Reliable sources of information include peer-reviewed medical journals, reputable health websites, and advice from healthcare professionals.

Quality and Dosage

The quality and dosage of herbal supplements can range widely between brands. It's important to choose supplements from reliable makers that adhere to good manufacturing practices (GMP) and provide clear labeling of ingredients and dosages. Be careful of supplements that make exaggerated or unsupported claims about their benefits.

Monitor Your Health

If you decide to try an alternative therapy, it's important to monitor your blood pressure and general health regularly. Keep track of any changes in your symptoms, blood pressure readings, or side effects. If you notice any negative effects, stop the therapy and consult your healthcare source immediately.

Alternative and complementary therapies, such as herbal supplements, acupuncture, massage, and mind-body practices, can play a supportive part in controlling high blood pressure.

However, they should be used in combination with, not as a replacement for, conventional treatments like medications and lifestyle changes. By working closely with your healthcare provider, you can build a comprehensive and personalized plan to manage your blood pressure and improve your overall health.

Remember, the key to good blood pressure management is a balanced method that combines the best of both traditional and alternative therapies.

Chapter 15: Working with Healthcare Providers

Building a Supportive Healthcare Team

Managing high blood pressure is a lifelong journey that requires a team of healthcare workers who understand your unique needs and can provide the best possible care. A supportive healthcare team is essential for effective blood pressure management, especially as you age and your health needs become more complex. This team can include a variety of professionals, each playing a distinct role in helping you maintain your health and avoid complications associated with hypertension.

Primary Care Physician (PCP)

Your primary care physician (PCP) is usually the first point of contact for controlling your blood pressure. They are responsible for conducting routine check-ups, prescribing medications, and monitoring your general health. Your PCP will measure your blood pressure readings, talk about lifestyle changes, and help you understand the importance of adhering to your treatment plan. They can also spot any potential issues early on and provide referrals to specialists if needed.

It's important to have a good relationship with your PCP, as they are the cornerstone of your healthcare team. Be open and honest about your symptoms, concerns, and any challenges you may face in controlling your blood pressure. Effective communication with your PCP can lead to better health results and a more personalized treatment plan.

Cardiologist

A cardiologist is an expert who focuses on heart health, including conditions like high blood pressure. If your blood pressure is particularly difficult to control, or if you have other cardiovascular problems, your PCP may send you to a cardiologist. This specialist can provide more in-depth analysis and treatment choices, such as advanced diagnostic tests, specialized medications, or procedures to manage your blood pressure and reduce the risk of heart disease.

Working with a cardiologist can be especially important if you have a family history of heart disease, have experienced heart-related symptoms, or have been labelled with conditions like atrial fibrillation or heart failure. A cardiologist will work closely with your PCP to ensure that your treatment plan is thorough and effective.

Dietitian or Nutritionist

Diet plays a critical role in managing blood pressure, and a registered dietitian or nutritionist can provide valuable advice on how to eat for better heart health. They can help you create a personalized eating plan that aligns with the Dietary Approaches to Stop Hypertension (DASH) diet or other heart-healthy dietary patterns.

A dietitian can also educate you on the importance of reducing sodium intake, raising potassium-rich foods, and incorporating other nutrients that support good blood pressure. They can provide useful tips for meal planning, grocery shopping, and dining out, making it easier to stick to your dietary goals.

Nurse Practitioner or Physician Assistant

Nurse practitioners (NPs) and physician assistants (PAs) are advanced practice providers who can play a significant part in managing your blood pressure. They often work alongside your PCP or specialist and are trained to perform many of the same tasks, such as performing physical exams, ordering tests, prescribing medications, and providing patient information.

NPs and PAs can offer extra support by answering your questions, helping you understand your treatment plan, and providing follow-up care. Their involvement can enhance the level of care you receive and ensure that you have access to timely and comprehensive healthcare services.

When to Consider a Specialist

While your primary care physician is usually your first resource for managing high blood pressure, there are times when visiting a specialist may be necessary. Specialists bring a higher level of expertise to specific areas of health, which can be crucial in managing more difficult or resistant cases of hypertension.

Signs You May Need a Specialist

1. Uncontrolled Blood Pressure: If your blood pressure stays high despite following your PCP's recommendations and taking prescribed medications, it may be time to see a specialist. Uncontrolled hypertension can lead to serious complications, and a specialist can help find underlying causes and offer advanced treatment choices.

2. Secondary Hypertension: In some cases, high blood pressure is caused by an underlying problem, such as kidney disease, hormonal disorders, or sleep apnea. This is known as secondary hypertension. If your PCP thinks that another condition is contributing to your high blood pressure, they may refer you to an appropriate specialist, such as a nephrologist (kidney specialist) or an endocrinologist (hormone specialist).

3. Complications from Hypertension: If you develop complications such as heart disease, stroke, or kidney damage, a specialist can provide the necessary care to manage these conditions and avoid further damage. For example, a nephrologist can help manage kidney-related problems, while a neurologist can address complications related to stroke or brain health.

4. Personal or Family History of Cardiovascular Disease: If you have a personal or family history of cardiovascular disease, a cardiologist can provide more specialized care to watch and manage your risk factors. Early intervention by a specialist can help avoid major heart-related complications.

Finding the Right Specialist

When considering a specialist, it's important to choose someone with the right knowledge and experience in managing hypertension and related conditions. Your PCP can provide suggestions and referrals to reputable specialists in your area. It's also important to ensure that the expert you choose is someone you feel comfortable with, as having a trusting relationship is key to effective care.

The Role of Pharmacists in Managing Your Blood Pressure

Pharmacists are often an underutilized resource in managing high blood pressure, but they play a crucial part in your healthcare team. Pharmacists are medication experts who can provide useful support in several ways:

Medication Management

One of the main roles of a pharmacist is to help manage your medications. This includes ensuring that you are taking the correct medications at the right amounts and that there are no harmful interactions between different drugs. Pharmacists can also provide information on how to take your medications properly, such as whether to take them with food or at a specific time of day.

If you experience side effects from your blood pressure medications, your pharmacist can offer help on how to manage them or suggest alternative medications that may have fewer side effects. They can also help you understand the importance of medication adherence and offer methods to help you remember to take your medications consistently.

Many pharmacies offer blood pressure monitoring services, which can be an easy way to keep track of your blood pressure between doctor visits. Some pharmacists are trained to take blood pressure readings and can provide instant feedback on whether your blood pressure is within a healthy range.

Pharmacists can also help you pick and use a home blood pressure monitor, ensuring that you are getting accurate readings. They can teach you how to properly measure your blood pressure at home and explain what your numbers mean.

Patient Education

Pharmacists are a great resource for patient instruction. They can provide advice on lifestyle changes that can help lower blood pressure, such as diet, exercise, and stress management. They can also offer advice on the use of over-the-counter medications and supplements, some of which can affect blood pressure.

For example, certain pain relievers, decongestants, and herbal supplements can raise blood pressure, so it's important to ask your pharmacist before using these products. Your pharmacist can help you choose safer options and ensure that any supplements you take are safe and compatible with your blood pressure medicines.

Medication Adherence Support

Taking your blood pressure medication as prescribed is important for managing your condition effectively. However, many people fight with medication adherence due to factors like forgetfulness, side effects, or complex dosing schedules. Pharmacists can give practical solutions to improve adherence, such as:

Medication Reminders: Pharmacists can suggest tools like pill organizers, medication reminder apps, or automatic refill services to help you stay on track with your medications.

Simplifying Medication Regimens: If you find it challenging to handle multiple medications, your pharmacist can work with your healthcare provider to simplify your regimen. This might involve combining medications into a single pill or changing dosing schedules to make it easier to remember.

Addressing Concerns: If you have concerns about your medications, such as fear of side effects or cost, your pharmacist can provide reassurance, offer solutions, or suggest lower-cost options.

Working with a healthcare team that includes a variety of professionals—such as your primary care physician, specialists, dietitians, nurse practitioners, and pharmacists—can significantly enhance your ability to control high blood pressure effectively.

Each member of your team plays a vital part in providing the comprehensive care you need to keep your health and prevent complications. By actively participating in your care, speaking freely with your healthcare providers, and utilizing the expertise of your healthcare team, you can take control of your blood pressure and improve your overall quality of life.

Chapter 16: Living with High Blood Pressure

Managing high blood pressure (hypertension) is a lifelong commitment that requires daily care and adaptation, especially as you age and your lifestyle changes. High blood pressure can greatly impact your overall health, but with the right strategies, you can keep it under control and continue living a full and active life. Below, we'll explore daily tips for managing blood pressure, how to adapt to changes as you age, and strategies for keeping your blood pressure while traveling.

Daily Tips for Managing Blood Pressure

1. Maintain a Heart-Healthy Diet

Your diet plays a key role in managing blood pressure. Incorporating heart-healthy foods into your daily meals can help reduce hypertension and lower the risk of problems.

- Follow the DASH Diet: The Dietary Approaches to Stop Hypertension (DASH) diet is specifically created to help reduce blood pressure. It emphasizes fruits, vegetables, whole grains, and lean proteins, and it suggests limiting sodium, saturated fat, and added sugars.

- Control Your Sodium Intake: High sodium intake is directly linked to higher blood pressure. Aim to eat less than 1,500 mg of sodium per day. Avoid prepared foods, which are often high in sodium, and use herbs and spices to flavor your meals instead of salt.

- Eat More Potassium-Rich Foods: Potassium can help balance the effects of sodium on blood pressure. Foods like bananas, oranges, spinach, and sweet potatoes are great sources of potassium.

- Limit Alcohol Consumption: Drinking alcohol can raise blood pressure, so it's important to consume it in limits. For most people, that means up to one drink per day for women and two drinks per day for men.

2. Stay Physically Active

Regular physical exercise is one of the most effective ways to manage high blood pressure. Exercise helps your heart become stronger and more efficient at pumping blood, which can lower the pressure on your arteries.

- Engage in Aerobic Exercise: Aim for at least 150 minutes of moderate-intensity aerobic exercise, such as brisk walking, swimming, or cycling, each week. If you're short on time, even shorter bursts of exercise, such as 10 minutes of walking, can be beneficial.

- Incorporate Strength Training: In addition to aerobic exercise, strength training exercises should be practiced at least two days per week. This can help lower blood pressure and improve overall cardiovascular health.

- Stay Active Throughout the Day: Sedentary behavior, such as sitting for long times, can negatively impact your blood pressure. Make an effort to stand up, stretch, and move around every hour, even if it's just for a few minutes.

3. *Monitor Your Blood Pressure at Home*

Regularly monitoring your blood pressure at home allows you to track your progress and make changes as needed. It also offers valuable information for your healthcare provider.

- Invest in a Reliable Blood Pressure Monitor: Choose an automated blood pressure monitor that is easy to use and has been approved for accuracy. Take readings at the same time each day, ideally in the morning before eating or taking medications.

- Keep a Blood Pressure Log: Record your readings in a blood pressure log, noting the date, time, and any things that might have affected the reading (e.g., stress, exercise). Share this log with your healthcare provider during your visits.

4. *Manage Stress Levels*

Chronic stress can contribute to high blood pressure, so it's important to find ways to manage it effectively.

- Practice Relaxation Techniques: Techniques like deep breathing exercises, meditation, and gradual muscle relaxation can help calm your mind and lower your blood pressure.

- Engage in Enjoyable Activities: Doing things you enjoy, such as reading, gardening, or spending time with loved ones, can help lower stress. Make time for these things every day.

- Get Enough Sleep: Poor sleep can boost stress levels and increase blood pressure. Aim for 7-8 hours of decent sleep each night. Establish a relaxing bedtime routine and keep a regular sleep schedule.

5. Avoid Tobacco and Limit Caffeine

Smoking is a major risk factor for high blood pressure and heart disease, while excessive caffeine intake can cause temporary spikes in blood pressure.

- Quit Smoking: If you smoke, quitting is one of the most important steps you can take to improve your blood pressure and general health. Seek help through smoking cessation programs, counseling, or medications if needed.

- Limit Caffeine Intake: Caffeine can raise blood pressure briefly, especially if you're sensitive to it. Pay attention to how caffeine affects you and try to limit your intake, especially from sources like coffee, tea, and energy drinks.

6. Adhere to Medication Prescriptions

If you've been prescribed medication for high blood pressure, it's crucial to take it as recommended. Medication adherence can greatly reduce the risk of heart attack, stroke, and other complications.

- Follow Your Prescription Schedule: Take your medication at the same time each day to keep consistent blood levels. If you have trouble remembering, set notes or use a pill organizer.
- Communicate with Your Doctor: If you experience side effects or have worries about your medication, talk to your doctor. They may change your dosage or switch you to a different medication.

Adapting to Changes as You Age

As you age, your body sees changes that can affect how you manage high blood pressure. Being aware of these changes and adjusting your approach can help you keep control over your blood pressure.

1. Monitor for New Symptoms

Aging can increase the chance of having other health conditions that affect blood pressure, such as diabetes, kidney disease, or vascular issues. Be vigilant about new symptoms, such as dizziness, blurred vision, or chest pain, and report them to your healthcare provider quickly.

2. Adjust Your Exercise Routine

While staying active is important at any age, older people may need to modify their exercise routines to accommodate physical limitations or chronic conditions.

- Opt for Low-Impact Activities: Low-impact exercises, such as swimming, walking, or using a stationary bike, can be easier on your joints while still offering cardiovascular benefits.
- Incorporate Balance and Flexibility Exercises: Balance exercises, such as tai chi or standing on one leg, can help avoid falls, while stretching can improve flexibility and reduce the risk of injury.

3. Reassess Your Diet

As metabolism slows with age, it's important to adjust your diet to avoid weight gain, which can raise blood pressure.

- Focus on Nutrient-Dense Foods: Choose foods that provide a high amount of nutrients compared to their calorie content. This includes fruits, veggies, lean proteins, and whole grains.
- Stay Hydrated: Older adults are at greater risk of dehydration, which can affect blood pressure. Drink plenty of water throughout the day, and limit sugary or caffeinated drinks.

4. Review Your Medications

The way your body processes medication can change with age, possibly requiring adjustments to your prescriptions.

- Regular Medication Reviews: Schedule regular reviews of your medicines with your healthcare provider to ensure that they are still appropriate for your needs. Your doctor may adjust dosages or suggest alternative treatments if necessary.

Traveling and Blood Pressure Management

Traveling can disrupt your regular routine, but with some planning, you can manage your blood pressure effectively while away from home.

1. Plan Ahead

Traveling often involves changes in diet, activity levels, and time zones, all of which can affect blood pressure.

● Pack Your Medications: Ensure you have enough medicine to last the entire trip, plus a few extra days' worth in case of delays. Carry your medication in your hand luggage so that it's always available.

● Plan for Meals: Research your destination and plan where you will eat to ensure you have access to healthy, low-sodium choices. If possible, pack some healthy snacks, such as nuts, veggies, or whole-grain crackers.

● Prepare for Time Zone Changes: If traveling across time zones, ask your doctor about how to adjust your medication schedule. Small shifts may be necessary to avoid disrupting your blood pressure control.

2. Stay Active During Travel

Long times of sitting, such as during flights or car rides, can negatively affect circulation and blood pressure.

- Move Regularly: Take stops to stand up, stretch, and walk around every hour during long trips. Simple exercises, like foot pumps or shoulder rolls, can also help keep circulation.

- Exercise at Your Destination: Incorporate physical exercise into your travel plans, whether it's a morning walk, a visit to a local park, or using the hotel gym. Staying busy will help keep your blood pressure in check.

3. Manage Stress and Sleep

Traveling can be stressful, and changes in habit can affect your sleep patterns, both of which can impact blood pressure.

- Practice Stress-Relief Techniques: Deep breathing, meditation, or listening to calming music can help lower stress during travel. These techniques can be especially helpful during stressful scenarios, such as delays or navigating unfamiliar places.

- Prioritize Sleep: Ensure you get proper rest while traveling. Stick to a regular sleep schedule as much as possible, and build a calming bedtime routine to help you unwind, even in an unfamiliar environment.

Managing high blood pressure requires daily attention and adjustments, especially as you age and encounter different life circumstances like travel.

Chapter 17: Preventing Complications

Managing high blood pressure is crucial because, if left unchecked, it can lead to serious and possibly life-threatening complications. These complications often affect vital organs like the heart, kidneys, and brain, which can significantly impact your general health and quality of life. Understanding how to protect these organs and reduce your chance of severe outcomes is key to properly managing high blood pressure.

Keeping Your Heart Healthy

High blood pressure, or hypertension, directly affects the heart by making it work harder to pump blood throughout the body. Over time, this increased workload can cause the heart muscle to thicken and stiffen, which may lead to different forms of heart disease.

1. The Link Between High Blood Pressure and Heart Disease

High blood pressure can damage the arteries that supply blood to your heart, making them less elastic and more prone to plaque buildup—a disease known as atherosclerosis. This buildup narrows the vessels and can lead to coronary artery disease, which is the most common cause of heart attacks.

Additionally, the constant pressure can cause the heart's walls to thicken, a disease known as left ventricular hypertrophy. This thickening makes it harder for the heart to pump efficiently, possibly leading to heart failure, where the heart can't pump enough blood to meet the body's needs.

2. *Heart-Healthy Habits*

To keep your heart healthy, it's important to adopt habits that reduce the strain on your cardiovascular system and promote overall heart health.

- Healthy Diet: A diet rich in fruits, veggies, whole grains, lean proteins, and low-fat dairy can help lower blood pressure and support heart health. Reducing salt intake is particularly important, as high sodium levels can cause your body to hold water, increasing blood pressure and the strain on your heart.
- Regular Exercise: Engaging in regular physical exercise strengthens the heart,

making it more efficient at pumping blood. Aim for at least 30 minutes of moderate activity most days of the week. Activities like walking, swimming, or cycling are great choices.

- Weight Management: Maintaining a healthy weight is important for heart health. Excess weight increases the strain on your heart and can lead to higher blood pressure. Even losing a small amount of weight can have a significant effect on lowering blood pressure and improving heart function.

- Avoid Smoking and Limit Alcohol: Smoking harms the blood vessels, increasing the risk of heart disease. Quitting smoking is one of the best things you can do for your heart. Additionally, limiting alcohol intake is important because excessive drinking can raise blood pressure and add to heart disease.

Protecting Your Kidneys

Your kidneys play a critical part in regulating blood pressure by controlling the balance of fluids and electrolytes in your body. High blood pressure can damage the blood vessels in the kidneys, leading to kidney disease, which further exacerbates hypertension in a dangerous loop.

1. The Connection Between Hypertension and Kidney Disease

High blood pressure can cause the small blood vessels in the kidneys to narrow and harden, lowering their ability to filter blood effectively. When the kidneys are damaged, they can't control blood pressure as well, leading to even higher blood pressure. This can finally lead to chronic kidney disease (CKD), where the kidneys gradually lose function.

In severe cases, CKD can move to end-stage renal disease (ESRD), where the kidneys fail completely and dialysis or a kidney transplant becomes necessary. High blood pressure is one of the leading causes of kidney failure, so protecting your kidneys is vital.

2. Strategies to Protect Your Kidneys

To protect your kidneys from the harmful effects of high blood pressure, it's important to manage your blood pressure and adopt kidney-friendly habits.

- Blood Pressure Control: Keeping your blood pressure within a healthy level is the most important step you can take to protect your kidneys. Regular monitoring and following your doctor's advice on medications and lifestyle changes are important.

- Healthy Diet: A kidney-friendly diet includes controlling your salt intake, as too much sodium can increase high blood pressure and strain your kidneys. Additionally, managing your intake of protein and potassium may be necessary if you have kidney disease, as recommended by your healthcare provider.

- Stay Hydrated: Drinking enough water is important for kidney health because it helps your kidneys filter waste from your blood. However, the amount of water you should drink varies depending on your health, so it's best to consult your doctor.

- Monitor Blood Sugar: If you have diabetes, managing your blood sugar levels is important because high blood sugar can damage the blood vessels in the kidneys, leading to diabetic nephropathy, a type of kidney disease.

Reducing the Risk of Stroke and Other Complications

Stroke is one of the most dangerous complications of high blood pressure. Hypertension can weaken and damage the blood vessels in the brain, increasing the chance of both ischemic (caused by a blockage) and hemorrhagic (caused by bleeding) strokes. Reducing the risk of stroke involves both managing your blood pressure and making lifestyle changes that protect your brain health.

1. How High Blood Pressure Increases Stroke Risk

When blood pressure is constantly high, it can lead to the formation of blood clots in the arteries that supply blood to the brain. If a clot stops blood flow to the brain, it can cause an ischemic stroke. On the other hand, high blood pressure can also cause blood vessels in the brain to burst, leading to a hemorrhagic stroke, which is often more dangerous and disabling.

Besides stroke, high blood pressure can also lead to other problems like aneurysms (weakened areas in blood vessel walls that can rupture) and vascular dementia, a type of cognitive decline caused by reduced blood flow to the brain.

2. Strategies to Reduce Stroke Risk

Preventing stroke and other complications from high blood pressure requires a mix of lifestyle changes and careful management of your condition.

- Monitor Blood Pressure Regularly: Regular monitoring helps you stay on top of your blood pressure levels and make changes as needed. Home tracking is a useful tool, and you should also have your blood pressure checked by your doctor regularly.

- Follow Medication Regimens: If your doctor has prescribed blood pressure medication, it's crucial to take it as told. Missing doses or stopping medicine can cause your blood pressure to spike, increasing the risk of a stroke.

- Adopt a Healthy Lifestyle: A balanced diet, regular exercise, not smoking, and limiting alcohol can all help lower your chance of stroke. Additionally, managing stress through relaxation techniques can also help to lower blood pressure.

- Recognize Stroke Warning Signs: Knowing the signs of a stroke can help you act quickly and seek emergency medical care, which is critical for minimizing damage. Signs include sudden numbness or weakness, especially on one side of the body, confusion, trouble speaking or understanding, difficulty seeing, dizziness, and strong headache.

Preventing complications from high blood pressure is important for maintaining a healthy, active life. By focusing on keeping your heart and kidneys healthy and lowering the risk of stroke, you can minimize the long-term effects of hypertension.

Chapter 18: The Role of Family and Caregivers

Managing high blood pressure is a lifelong responsibility, especially as we age. The support of family and caregivers can play a crucial role in helping to maintain a healthy lifestyle, stick to treatment plans, and deal with the challenges that come with managing a chronic condition. Involving loved ones, creating a supportive home environment, and effectively communicating your needs are essential steps in ensuring successful blood pressure control and overall well-being.

Involving Loved Ones in Your Care

One of the most important aspects of managing high blood pressure is ensuring that you have a good support system. Involving family members and caregivers in your care can make a major difference in how well you manage your condition. Loved ones can offer mental support, help with daily tasks, and encourage you to stick to your treatment plan.

1. Sharing Information

Educating your family about high blood pressure is the first step in involving them in your care. This includes explaining what high blood pressure is, how it affects your body, and why it's important to control it. Share with them the details of your treatment plan, including any medicines you're taking, dietary restrictions, and the importance of regular exercise. The more they understand about your condition, the better equipped they'll be to help you.

2. Encouragement and Motivation

Living with high blood pressure often requires making major lifestyle changes, such as adopting a healthier diet, increasing physical activity, and managing stress. These changes can be challenging to keep on your own, but with the encouragement and support of loved ones, they become more manageable. Family members can help motivate you to stay on track with your health goals, whether it's by joining you for daily walks, preparing healthy meals together, or learning relaxation techniques as a group.

3. Monitoring and Reminders

Family members and caregivers can also assist with monitoring your blood pressure and telling you to take your medications. Regular monitoring is crucial for tracking your progress and ensuring that your blood pressure stays within a healthy range. Loved ones can help by learning how to use a home blood pressure monitor and keeping a log of your numbers. They can also tell you to take your medication at the correct times, which is especially important if you have a complex medication regimen.

Creating a Supportive Home Environment

A supportive home environment is important for managing high blood pressure successfully. Your living space should support healthy habits and make it easier for you to stick to your treatment plan. By making small changes to your home and daily routine, you can create an environment that supports your health and well-being.

1. Diet and Nutrition Support

One of the key aspects of controlling high blood pressure is following a healthy diet, such as the DASH (Dietary Approaches to Stop Hypertension) diet, which emphasizes fruits, vegetables, whole grains, and low-fat dairy products while reducing sodium intake. Family members can help by ensuring that the home is stocked with healthy foods and by sharing in meal planning and preparation. This not only makes it easier to stick to your dietary goals but also develops a sense of teamwork and shared responsibility.

For instance, loved ones can help by reading food labels to check for sodium content, finding recipes that match with your dietary needs, and encouraging everyone in the household to eat healthier. This collective method ensures that you don't feel isolated in your dietary changes and that everyone benefits from healthier eating habits.

2. Encouraging Physical Activity

Physical exercise is another crucial component of managing high blood pressure. Incorporating regular exercise into your daily routine can help lower blood pressure and improve general heart health. Family members can play a significant role in this by joining you in physical activities, such as walks, swimming, or even gardening.

Creating a home environment that encourages physical exercise can also be helpful. For example, designating a particular area in your home for exercise, such as a space for yoga or stretching, can make it easier to incorporate physical activity into your daily routine. Loved ones can also join in group activities or outings that involve physical exercise, making it a fun and social experience rather than a chore.

Chronic stress can significantly impact blood pressure, so having a calm and stress-free environment at home is important. Family members can help by being mindful of the stressors in your surroundings and working together to reduce them. This might involve setting aside time each day for relaxation, practicing stress-reducing activities together (such as meditation or deep breathing exercises), or simply ensuring that the home is a peaceful and supportive place.

If stress is caused by specific factors, such as financial concerns or family conflicts, addressing these issues openly and working together to find solutions can help lower overall stress levels. Open communication and a willingness to work together are key to building a supportive environment that supports relaxation and well-being.

Communicating Your Needs

Effective communication with your family and caregivers is important for managing high blood pressure successfully. Being open and honest about your wants, concerns, and challenges can help ensure that you receive the support you require. It also allows your loved ones to better understand how they can help you in managing your condition.

1. Expressing Your Needs Clearly

It's important to be clear and direct when expressing your needs to your family and caregivers. This includes discussing any physical limitations you may have, such as difficulty with certain jobs or needing help with medication management. By expressing your wants openly, you allow your loved ones to step in and offer assistance where it's most needed.

For example, if you're feeling overwhelmed by the dietary changes needed to manage your blood pressure, let your family know that you could use help with meal planning or grocery shopping. If you find it challenging to stay inspired with exercise, ask a loved one to join you for daily walks or workouts. Clear communication ensures that your support system can provide the help you need when you need it.

2. Discussing Challenges and Concerns

Living with high blood pressure can be difficult, and it's normal to experience moments of frustration, fear, or uncertainty. Sharing these feelings with your loved ones can help relieve some of the emotional load and allow your support system to offer encouragement and reassurance.

For instance, if you're afraid about the side effects of a new medication or the difficulty of sticking to your treatment plan, talk about these concerns with your family. They may be able to offer a viewpoint, help you explore solutions, or simply provide a listening ear. Openly discussing your challenges also helps your loved ones understand the emotional and mental aspects of handling high blood pressure, allowing them to offer more effective support.

3. Setting Boundaries

While it's important to involve family members in your care, it's equally important to set boundaries to keep your independence and avoid feelings of being overwhelmed. Setting boundaries ensures that your loved ones understand how and when you prefer to receive support and that you keep control over your own health decisions.

For example, you might ask family members to remember you about your medication but request that they respect your privacy during doctor's appointments. Or you might respect help with meal preparation but prefer to exercise alone. Communicating these preferences clearly can help avoid misunderstandings and ensure that the support you receive aligns with your needs.

Chapter 19: Tools and Apps for Blood Pressure Management

Managing high blood pressure effectively takes a combination of lifestyle changes, regular monitoring, and staying informed about your health. In today's digital age, technology has made it easier than ever to keep track of your blood pressure, stay motivated, and access useful resources for support. Tools like mobile apps, wearable devices, and online platforms can play a vital role in helping you keep control over your blood pressure and overall health. This section explores some of the best apps, wearable devices, and online tools available for managing high blood pressure.

Best Apps for Monitoring and Managing Blood Pressure

Mobile apps have become indispensable tools for many people controlling chronic conditions, including high blood pressure. These apps offer a range of features that make it easier to track your blood pressure readings, watch trends over time, and stay on top of your health goals. Here are some of the best apps available for blood pressure management:

1. Blood Pressure Monitor by MedM

MedM's Blood Pressure Monitor app is a simple yet powerful tool for checking your blood pressure. It allows you to log your readings manually or import data straight from compatible devices. The app also offers customizable reminders to help you stay on plan with your monitoring. One of its key features is the ability to create detailed reports, which can be shared with your healthcare provider. This makes it easier to track your progress and make informed choices about your treatment plan.

2. *My Blood Pressure by Hypertension Canada*

My Blood Pressure is an app created by Hypertension Canada, specifically designed for individuals managing high blood pressure. It offers a user-friendly interface for logging blood pressure readings, setting reminders for medication, and accessing educational resources. The app also includes features like goal setting and personalized tips based on your readings, helping you stay motivated and informed about your situation.

3. Heartify: Heart Health Monitor

Heartify is a complete heart health app that goes beyond just blood pressure tracking. It offers features for monitoring various parts of cardiovascular health, including heart rate, stress levels, and physical activity. The app uses data from wearable devices to provide a holistic view of your heart health, making it a valuable tool for those who want to take a proactive approach to controlling high blood pressure. Heartify also offers insights and tips based on your data, helping you make lifestyle changes that can improve your blood pressure and general well-being.

4. Qardio Heart Health

Qardio Heart Health is another great app for managing blood pressure. It connects with

Qardio's range of health devices, including blood pressure monitors, to automatically record and analyze your results. The app offers detailed graphs and charts that help you understand your blood pressure trends over time. It also features reminders for taking measurements and medicines, making it easier to stick to your management plan.

Additionally, Qardio Heart Health allows you to share your data with your healthcare provider, facilitating better conversation and personalized care.

Wearable Devices and How They Can Help

Wearable devices have revolutionized the way we track our health. These gadgets offer constant tracking of various health metrics, including blood pressure, heart rate, and physical activity levels. For individuals with high blood pressure, wearables can be especially beneficial in providing real-time data and alerts that help avoid complications. Here are some of the most useful wearable gadgets for managing blood pressure:

1. Smartwatches with Blood Pressure Monitoring

Several smartwatches now offer blood pressure tracking features, allowing you to check your blood pressure at any time without the need for a traditional cuff. Devices like the Samsung Galaxy Watch and Fitbit Sense come packed with sensors that measure blood pressure through pulse wave analysis. These watches also track your heart rate, sleep patterns, and physical activity, giving a comprehensive view of your cardiovascular health. The convenience of having all this data on your wrist makes it easier to stay informed and take action when required.

2. Wearable Blood Pressure Monitors

Wearable blood pressure monitors, such as the Omron HeartGuide, offer medical-grade accuracy in a portable version. These devices are meant to be worn like a regular watch but have built-in cuffs that inflate to take precise blood pressure readings. The data is then synced to a companion app, where you can review your numbers, set reminders, and track trends over time. Wearable monitors are particularly useful for individuals who need to check their blood pressure frequently or those who want to track their readings throughout the day.

3. Fitness Trackers with Health Monitoring Features

Fitness trackers like the Apple Watch, Garmin Vivosmart, and Whoop Strap have grown beyond simple step counters. Many now include tools for tracking heart rate variability, sleep quality, and stress levels, all of which are important for managing high blood pressure. While these devices may not provide blood pressure readings as accurately as medical-grade monitors, they offer important insights into your overall health. By keeping track of your physical activity, sleep, and stress, you can make informed choices that positively impact your blood pressure management.

Online Resources for Education and Support

In addition to apps and wearables, online resources can provide useful education and support for managing high blood pressure. These platforms offer access to expert advice, community support, and the latest research, helping you stay informed and inspired. Here are some of the best online tools for blood pressure management:

1. American Heart Association (AHA)

The American Heart Association is one of the main sources of information on cardiovascular health, including high blood pressure. Their website offers a wealth of resources, from educational papers and videos to tools for tracking your blood pressure and managing your condition. The AHA also offers guidelines on diet, exercise, and medication adherence, making it a complete resource for anyone looking to improve their heart health.

2. Hypertension Canada

Hypertension Canada's website is a great resource for individuals managing high blood pressure. It gives detailed information on the causes, symptoms, and treatment of hypertension, along with tips for lifestyle changes that can help lower blood pressure. The site also features a section dedicated to patient tools, including guides on how to measure blood pressure properly, how to choose the right medications, and how to reduce sodium intake. Additionally, Hypertension Canada offers access to webinars and support groups, allowing you to connect with experts and others who share your condition.

3. Mayo Clinic's Hypertension Resources

The Mayo Clinic is renowned for its expertise in medical care, and its online tools on hypertension are no exception. The Mayo Clinic's website offers in-depth information on high blood pressure, including its causes, risk factors, and treatment choices. You can also find practical tips for managing your condition, such as help on diet, exercise, and stress reduction. The site's interactive tools, such as symptom checkers and medication guides, make it easier to understand and control your health.

4. Patient Advocacy and Support Groups

Online forums and support groups can be useful for individuals living with high blood pressure. Platforms like HealthUnlocked, PatientsLikeMe, and the American Heart Association's Support Network offer communities where you can connect with others who are having similar challenges. These groups provide a space for sharing experiences, asking questions, and getting emotional support. Being part of a community can help you feel less isolated and more powerful in your journey to manage high blood pressure.

Conclusion

Managing high blood pressure is a lifelong journey, but it's one that you can navigate successfully with the right mindset, tools, and support. As you've learned throughout this guide, controlling blood pressure involves more than just taking medication—it's about adopting a comprehensive approach that includes healthy eating, regular physical activity, stress management, and consistent monitoring.

It's important to remember that progress might be gradual, and setbacks can happen. However, each positive change you make contributes to a healthier heart and a better quality of life. For instance, incorporating the DASH diet or reducing your sodium intake might seem challenging at first, but over time, these adjustments can become second nature, leading to significant improvements in your blood pressure and overall well-being. Similarly, if you begin a new exercise routine, it may take some time before you notice changes in your blood pressure, but consistency will yield results.

You are not alone in this journey. Support from loved ones, healthcare providers, and even technology can make a significant difference. Engaging with a healthcare team that understands your needs and can provide personalized advice is crucial. Additionally, leveraging tools like mobile apps, wearable devices, and online communities can help you stay on track and feel supported.

Most importantly, don't underestimate the power of small, steady steps. Every effort you make—whether it's a short walk, a healthier meal choice, or a moment of meditation—adds up to a healthier you. Celebrate each victory, no matter how small, and use it as motivation to keep moving forward.

Final Thoughts on Living Well with High Blood Pressure

Living with high blood pressure does not mean you have to live in fear or anxiety about your health. Instead, it can be an opportunity to take control of your life and make choices that enhance your well-being. This guide has provided you with a range of strategies, from dietary adjustments and exercise routines to stress management techniques and medication adherence. The goal is not just to lower your blood pressure numbers, but to improve your overall quality of life.

Understanding that blood pressure management is a long-term commitment is key. It's not about making drastic changes overnight, but rather about incorporating sustainable habits that you can maintain over time. For example, if you've learned to enjoy healthier foods, discovered a new exercise you love, or found effective ways to relax, you're not just managing your blood pressure—you're improving your life in countless other ways.

It's also essential to stay informed and proactive about your health. Keep up with regular check-ups, monitor your blood pressure at home, and stay connected with your healthcare team. Remember that your health is dynamic, and what works for you today may need to be adjusted as you age or as your life circumstances change. Be open to learning and adapting as you go.

In conclusion, living well with high blood pressure is entirely possible with the right approach. By staying committed to the strategies outlined in this guide—healthy eating, regular physical activity, stress management, medication adherence, and routine monitoring—you can maintain a healthy blood pressure and enjoy a fulfilling life. This journey is about more than just managing a condition; it's about embracing a lifestyle that promotes long-term health and happiness.

Take each day as it comes, make the best choices you can, and remember that every positive step you take brings you closer to a healthier, happier life.